IN SEARCH OF CIRCLE Z

Constance Dry

In Search of Circle Z

MIGRAINE, MEMORYSCAPES, AND DIORAMAS

PAUL DRY BOOKS

Philadelphia 2023

First Paul Dry Books Edition, 2023

Paul Dry Books, Inc.
Philadelphia, Pennsylvania
www.pauldrybooks.com

ISBN: 978-1-58988-180-8

Printed in the United States of America

Library of Congress Control Number: 2023942491

CONTENTS

TO MIRA

Mira, I see you sitting there across from me in this crowded waiting room. You are so ragged and disheveled, all bent over upon yourself, your neck barely supported by the small pillow you clutch. The grimace on your face reveals how much pain you suffer and how much energy it has consumed. The others here look withdrawn and ill as well, but they still give the impression of belonging to this temporary community of patients. You do not.

In all the times I have sat in this waiting room, I have never seen anyone quite like you. This book is about making, not just enduring. The memoryscapes I will describe became my way to gain momentary control over pain. They are powerful engines of production that morphed into ways of seeing that have produced many new experiences. Like you, all aspects of my life have been affected by migraine.

One early morning in August of 2021, I found myself sitting before an ancient apple tree set beside a section of the old acequia madre, or irrigation ditch, in Santa Fe. I thought of you again, Mira, imagining you this time in a different setting outside the waiting room of the Jefferson Headache Center in Philadelphia. The apple tree's branches bear tiny yellow apples that every now and then make a brief snapping sound when they hit the brick patio underneath the tree. High above, small birds dart among the branches of the trees that form a backdrop to the apple tree, and above them all, morning light sharpens as the brisk air warms. This is my speed. There are many times during a day I wish I could tolerate more noise, more activity, more engagement, because by nature I am not reclusive, but viewing this apple tree and the morning movement of the birds is just about the right amount of stimulation I can take. My internal gyroscope, so often askew, spins now in perfect balance. I engage with it using the hand I was dealt and I wish that for you as well.

CHAPTER ONE

IN THE MUSEUM

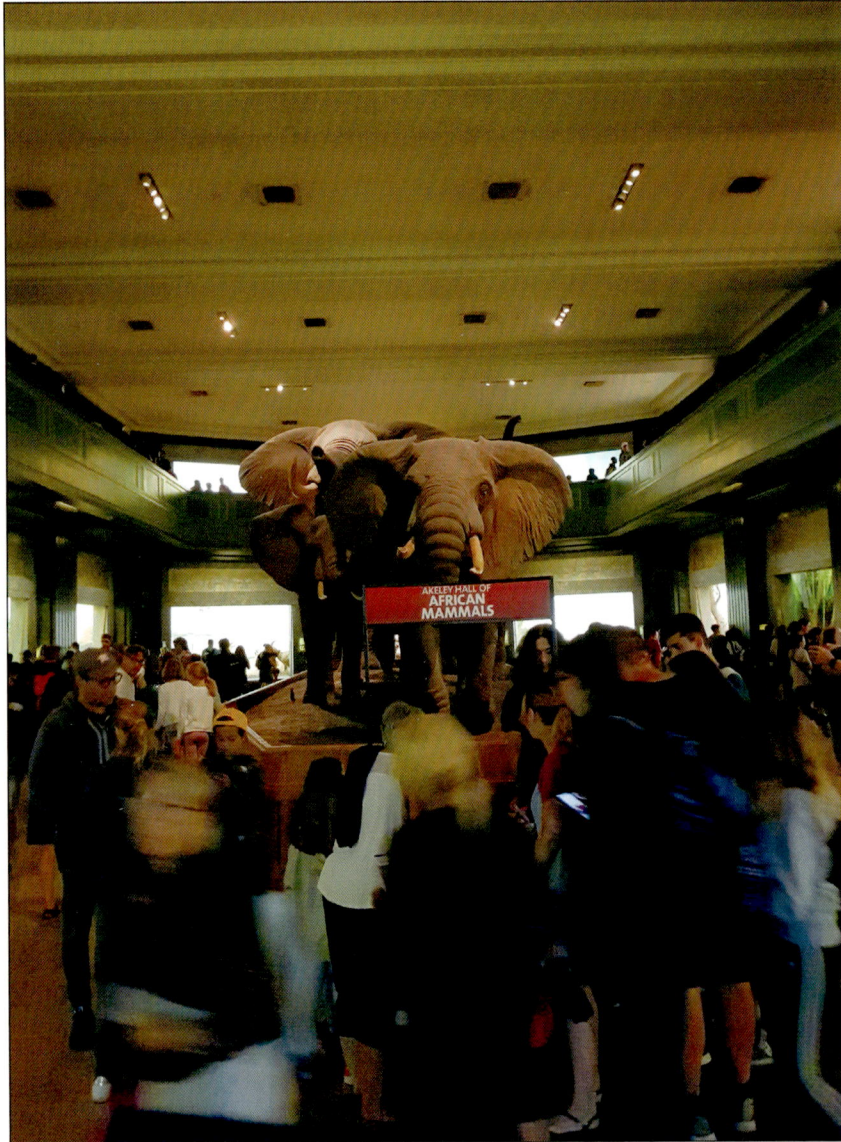

The Swirling Crowd, Akeley Hall of African Mammals,
American Museum of Natural History

A young girl, about seven years old, reaches up to grasp her mother's hand. She presses her other hand against the slanted plate glass window that encloses the Lion Diorama in the American Museum of Natural History in New York. Speaking loudly above the noise of the crowd, she asks, as many children here do, "Momma, are they real?" Turning toward the glass, she adds, "I'd like to be under those trees in there with them." The pride of five African lions on the other side almost touch the window. A resting female in the foreground licks her forearm. Behind her, a male with ample mane stands erect and looks outward towards us with an indirect, non-threatening gaze. The three remaining females fan out around him with ears alert and eyes attentive to any movement in the savannah beyond. The morning sun brightens the acres of kangaroo grass that match the color of the lions' hides. This imposing pride rests in the shade of a mulberry tree. Against the surrounding darkness of the Hall, the entire life-size diorama glows in its bronze frame. It is not alone, though; twenty-seven other dioramas line the walls. Each one invites many restless viewers to move on and take a look, and they all do.

I'm here too, standing in the crowd behind the mother and her daughter. All around me, dancing pinpricks of white light flash and flicker and for a moment briefly illuminate the faces that surround me. Many people in the moving crowd break stride to hold up their cellphones, press the button, and get the shots. They quickly record many dioramas in this way. I begin to walk among them, moving closer to the mother and child. As I walk through the flashes in the darkness, I recall a story once circulated about Native Americans in the West at the end of the nineteenth century who did not want their photographs taken because they believed that the camera and its images stole their souls and, in doing so, disrespected the spirit world. What, then, of the photographers here around me? What of their souls? What do they part with in this rapid, compulsive snapping of pictures? The mother and her daughter standing close to the glass window are camera-less. Their eyes alone register what they are seeing. They lean in and become more and more absorbed. They talk to each other and look through the plate glass and begin to point. Time passes. I step back again to better see them and the diorama at the same time. They linger and so do I. We create three fixed points in the swirling crowd.

I turn and walk back through the crowd toward a wooden bench in the center of the Hall. The bench encircles a coffin-shaped base with a herd of life-sized elephants rising above it. Eight of them, including mothers and a baby, move forward in agitated readiness toward the entrance to the two-story Carl Akeley Hall of African Mammals. Unlike the dioramas, the herd is unlit. The aroused elephants present a massive, dark, anchoring counterpoint to the two stories of dioramas that surround them. I sit down on the curved bench and look into the darkness and the crowd between the elephants and the dioramas. Seated next to me, four nannies chatter away. The charges at their feet sleep upright in parked strollers. Their unzipped down snowsuits bulge around them, not needed now on this warmer early spring day. Their caregivers often make this bench an afternoon stopping off place, convenient for gossip and naps. As I slump down into the heat of my own down jacket, the forms in the moving crowd in front of me begin to blur. I look up and see the mother and child move on to the next diorama. As I begin to doze again, the Lion Diorama becomes a smudge of light. The darkness of the moving crowd creates the visual sensation of a flicker as it interrupts the view of the lighted diorama cases. I nod off briefly, in the noise, behind the crowd, enveloped by the darkness. Half-asleep, I am partly here in the hall where I find myself and partly there, deep in the quiet of the savannah morning among the preening lions.

At my feet, a baby's cry startles me. I return to this spectacular interior space. It is itself, dioramas and interior space, its own place. Every inch of it has been designed for the purpose of looking. From where I sit behind the moving crowd, the eighteen-foot-high cases set within the walls glow like stop action film frames of the African vistas. Each presents a new scene with its own viewing point. When seen at a glance like this, they look like connected stills knitted together by the intervening dark spaces between them and the similar height of their horizons within.

These beautiful, immersive three-dimensional dioramas now bring to my mind a series of mental images of my own making that I have named "memoryscapes." Sitting here in the darkness, looking at the line of dioramas, I realize how much the memoryscapes have provided experiences similar to my viewing of dioramas. The memoryscapes appeared before my closed eyes. They looked like static still frames covering my vision, irresistible images of alluring beauty. These uncalled for images emerged spontaneously, rising from somewhere not immediately available to my memory, during a six-month period of pain following the onset, on October 2, 2003, of what was then thought to be viral meningitis. After this severe flu-like illness I was left with a painful continuous migraine that produced many alarming disruptions in my visual field during attacks. It took a number of visits to different specialists to determine that the pain I was experiencing was from a migraine that would not resolve. From that day forward, my seventeen years as a filmmaker ended, as I could no longer tolerate editing moving images or the audio of the sound track or the sound of music. I was nearing my sixtieth birthday.

The surprising, spontaneous images I named memory-scapes were in every way distinct from the other visual symptoms accompanying my chronic migraines. During a migraine I would attempt to hold these images in my mind's eye. Once I was familiar with them, I tried to capture their essence in drawings and constructions. Both their form as pictorial views and their content derived from the landscape of a particular place in the external world that I knew well: a ranch in Arizona that I have visited since childhood. There they rested, sidetracked, hidden and shelved in a dormant corner of my memory until the onset of migraine disease. Then, in a period of continuing pain, these hidden landscape bits surfaced and were presented to me in all their dazzling beauty. In time they seemed to migrate outward toward a shared visual experience with the great habitat dioramas in New York, their counterparts in the three-dimensional world.

This book traces the ways memoryscapes altered my experience of migraine pain, first through the mental re-construction and employment of these images during the initial six months of intense pain and then through my ongoing use of them in tandem with viewing dioramas as both became sources of visual enrichment and discovery.

Memoryscapes and dioramas became places of refuge, a source of neurological stabilization, and multi-layered experiences of wonder. In the years that followed the onset of chronic migraine disease, I made repeated visits to the sites at Circle Z Ranch where the memoryscapes emerged. I photographed these sites, then I drew the memoryscapes to show how they differed from the actual sites, and finally I tried to describe them in words, which proved to be the least satisfying. Back in Philadelphia, I constructed the memoryscapes as mini-dioramas and visited the New York dioramas, where I began to understand how similar the memoryscapes and dioramas were to each other as objects of beauty and refuge.

The four memoryscapes that appeared to my mind's eye were entirely different from the zig-zags, flashes, bursts, smudges, lines, and other visual interruptions I saw during a migraine. Today, twenty years after the onset of migraine disease, I find myself again in the Akeley Hall, re-entering the world of habitat dioramas to see what new experience I will have. Among the resting lions I will use my memory of past experiences here, my powers of observation, and my imagination. What I see within the refuge of each diorama differs every time I come but is always grounded in each dazzling scene, just as what I experience each time I call up a memoryscape in times of migraine pain is anchored in its specific landscape.

Like me, the mother and child view the Lion Diorama in a manner that cannot be achieved with the click of a cell phone camera. They take their time at each diorama, captivated by what they see because there is more and more to see. They are seeing a place in all three dimensions, a viewing experience unattainable through film or photography. When compared to this three-dimensional encounter, cell phone images become more like a form of note taking for remembered experiences, compressing and flattening space.

In front of me, the Lion Diorama recreates a real place, the Serengeti plain, east of Victoria in Africa, at a specific time on a specific day. It embodies a unique combination of scientific rendering and artistic illusion that is so dense in accurate detail that it equally convinces and engages the seven-year-old viewer, the botanist or businessman, or me of its veracity. Up close, each plant, each detail on the fur of the lion's back, is sensually satisfying and scientifically accurate. At the same time, when the diorama is viewed in its entirety, it is convincing as a real habitat. Each viewing yields new sights for the eye, just as if the viewer were scanning the landscape like a member of the pride.

Perhaps the mother standing there may have been on a safari to these very same African plains or perhaps she has never traveled much farther than the distance between her Brooklyn borough and the museum. It is likely that her daughter is already familiar with lions from having seen National Geographic specials. She may even have seen the giant neon lion in the ad for the Broadway play *The Lion King* above Times Square one day when she emerged from the subway with her mother after a visit to the Bronx Zoo. Most likely, they have just come from the Hall of Biodiversity here in the museum, where they have wandered along the walkway and peered into the Dzanga-Sangha rain forest to observe a herd of African elephants caught on film as they approach a distant waterhole at dawn. Each of these experiences produces its own form of visual engagement. None provides the same human scale or the prolonged, visual immersion that looking into the Lion Diorama yields. In the Akeley Hall, they can observe at their own pace, think their thoughts and conjure up a story while maintaining a spatial presence in a scene that seems so real it subverts their knowledge of its artificiality.

Today the act of absorbing this scene of resting lions, which I now share with the mother and her child, is repeated over and over by visitors who take the time to stop and linger. What is happening here for each of us is confirmation of what A.E. Parr, director of the museum at the height of the museum's initial commitment to dioramas in the early twentieth century, believed the primary function of natural history museums to be. They were to serve "as mental activators and catalysts rather than didactic communicators of knowledge."[1] Understood this way, the habitat dioramas bridge the traditional divide between science and art. They do this by creating the perception of deep atmospheric space and realistic detail. Within the credible interior space of the diorama we view the animal specimens in life-like poses, embedded in their natural habitat. We stand next to the lions at eye-level, measuring our size directly against theirs for as long as we wish.

The mother and child have moved on, so I rise from the bench and move toward the diorama to stand where they stood. I visually and imaginatively pass through the clear, reflection-free plate glass and settle into an open space in the middle of the pride in the foreground. Forming a protective perimeter around me, the five lions shelter me and look outward. In this refuge I sit among them, safe in this fixed moment. The Lion Diorama, like all the habitat dioramas with taxidermied animals, suggests a drama. Here, two of the females keep their eyes on possible prey, a distant herd of antelopes and wildebeests. As I look outward, the savannah opens to me in ever-expanding detail: the grasses, the slope of the land, the trees, the herds all interconnect to create the habitat for this pride of lions. I have taken refuge here among them on a number of visits before today. I have crouched low to the ground beyond them, enveloped by the grasses. Hidden this way, I have looked out over the savannah, trying to approximate their sight lines. Today, I notice the profusion of violet flowers on a low bush. And from that bush I move farther out onto the unrolling savannah, far from New York, into the middle distance where the morning sun lends a distinct sweet smell to the warming earth and the swirling insects rise around me.[2]

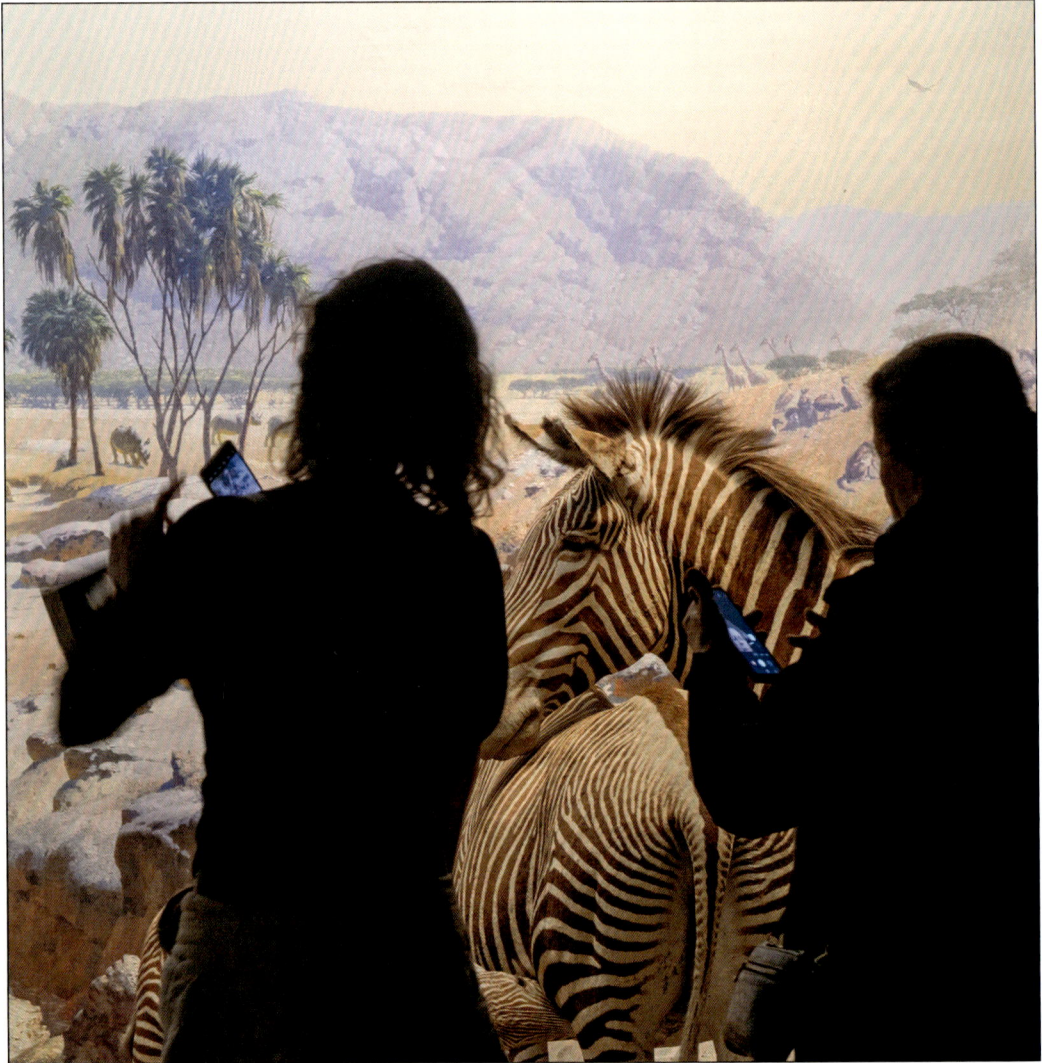

Cell Phones and Zebras, Akeley Hall of African Mammals,
American Museum of Natural History

Justin Audet

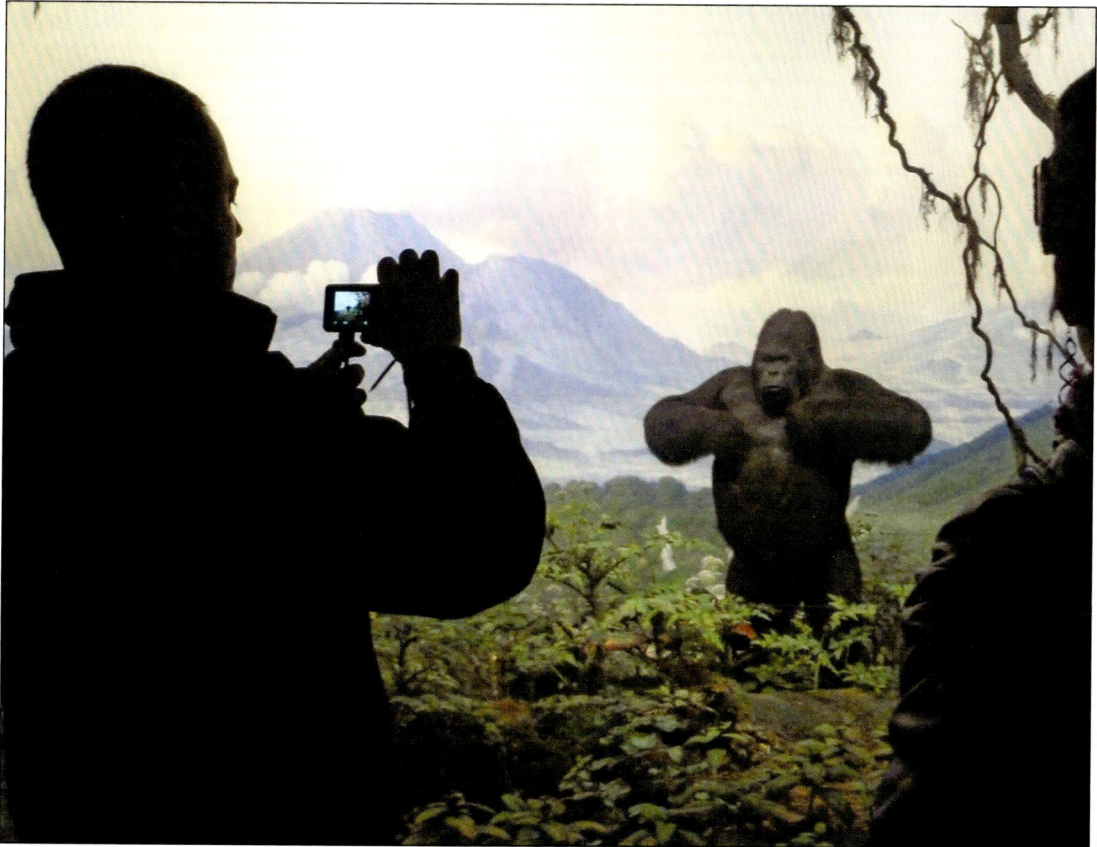

Photographing the Gorilla, Akeley Hall

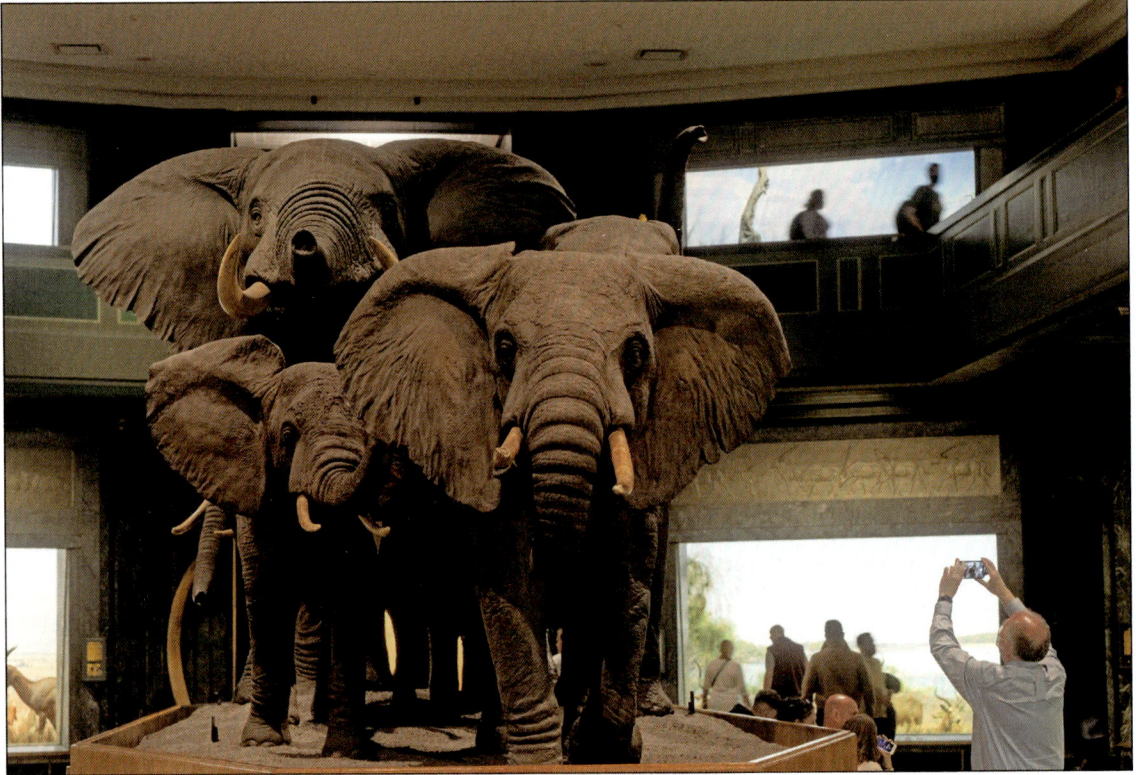

Getting the Shot, Akeley Hall

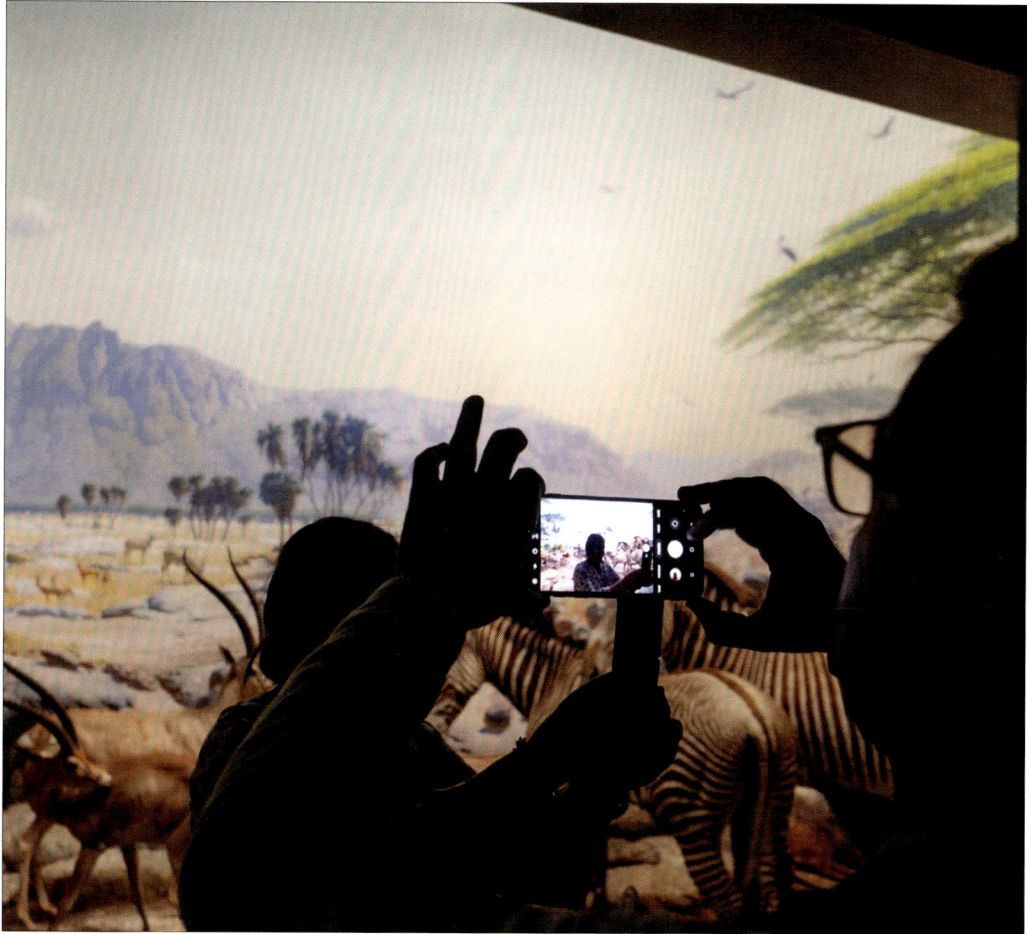

Shots of Selfies in Akeley Hall

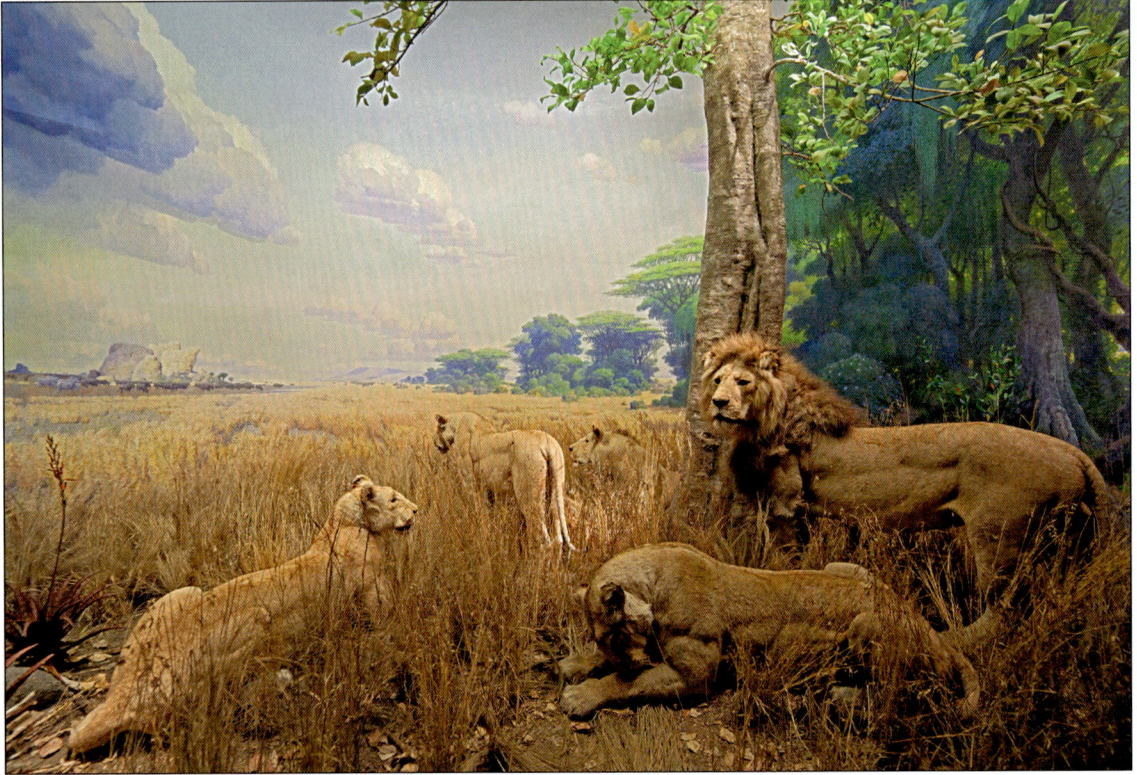

Lion Diorama, Akeley Hall

IN THE MOVIE THEATER

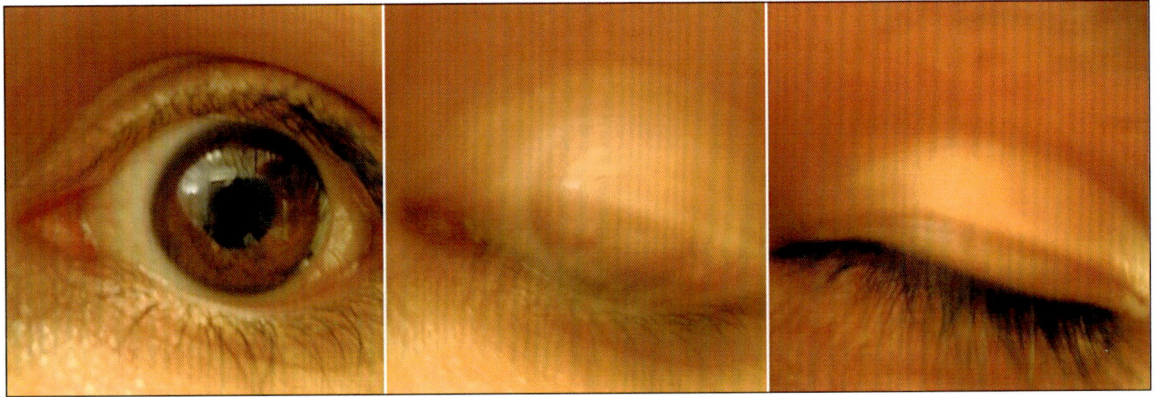

The Blink of an Eye

I settle into my seat in the nearly empty Ritz 5 movie theater to wait for the noon film to begin. Here there is no proscenium arch or protruding stage up front or heavy curtain, as there was in the old Jeffery Theater of my 1950s Chicago childhood. The Jeffery, opened in 1925, designed by William P. Doerr, was an ornate, neo-classical theater built to host vaudeville acts requiring a curtained stage. When it was converted to a movie theater in the late twenties, it began its more enduring life with the addition of a screen and projection booth housed on the balcony level. Located on a booming commercial strip on Chicago's South Side, it seated almost 1,800. Unaccompanied by my parents, on Saturday afternoons I walked from 69th to 71st Street to the movie theater with my sister. There, I sat mesmerized by the distant images and how they merged into one another on the giant screen. My vision was poor and the huge pictures showed me things I had trouble seeing in real life. Image usurped story by a long shot.

Today, I look at a simple, blank movie screen. It floats free in front of me, beyond the curving rows of seats here in the small theater in Philadelphia. In the quiet before the trailers begin, I sink back into the thick cushion of my reclining seat and relax in the darkness surrounding me. After a minute, I close my eyes. The screen's linen-like white surface is just as smooth as the unruffled surface that I see when I close my eyes. In the comforting silence I continue to savor the blankness on the inner surface of my mind's eye. Right now, these two screens, the external movie screen and the internal screen, appear to be duplicates. When I blink to compare the outer with the inner, I become aware of the absence of any mark or image on either surface. Neither one suggests any indication of depth or internal orientation. Their empty expanses provide smooth visual backgrounds onto which completely formed images, as well as shadings of light, may or may not attach themselves. Each of my involuntary blinks interrupts the appearance of the movie screen with the appearance of this unusually calm internal screen. As I perceive them in this quiet moment, outer and inner screens match. For most of my life I took it for granted that the outer world and my mind's eye were neurologically attuned with one another.

For most of us, images appear on the internal screen of our mind's eye; some are after-images, some come from dreams, others emerge out of memory, but in addition other ones have also appeared to me as a consequence of severe migraines and memoryscapes. These visual interruptions are either the product of the migraines themselves, in the form of auras and visual phosphenes, or they are fully-formed, self-sustaining memoryscapes. When I close my eyes during a migraine, I can see one or the other. Now, here in the Ritz 5 theater, migraine-free, eyes closed and eyes open, both the inner screen of my mind's eye and the outer movie screen are unmarked canvases awaiting the imprint of an image. The shadow-less dim light, the silence, the lack of movement, all soothe my senses. I relax and feel as if I am suspended in a motionless pool of supportive water. Because of migraine disease, I live with the awareness that the boundaries between the inner screen of my mind's eye and the images I receive from the outer world, which I once assumed were stable and separate, are in fact permeable. What I see with my eyes closed and what I see with my eyes open are at times both overlaid with disturbing neurological eruptions during a migraine.

In 1926, Friedrich Kiesler, a Viennese architect, set designer, and artist, emigrated to America to become part of the modernist design movement in New York that emphasized functionalism in architecture and art. At the same time as the Jeffery Theater was being built in Chicago, Kiesler designed a new kind of theater, the sole purpose of which was the projection of movies. His movie theater, the Film Guild Cinema, was built in Greenwich Village in 1929, just one year after the release of the first talking movie, *The Jazz Singer.* In his innovative design, Kiesler eliminated the entire proscenium and surrounding ornamentation that comprised the vaudeville stage. Having removed the traditional elements of the fourth wall separating the audience from the screen, Kiesler's design invited the audience to a far more direct viewing of moving pictures.

In the narrow Guild Theater the viewer faced forward to see the outline of a large black circle set on a white square wall at the front of the theater. This circle evokes a floor-to-ceiling rounded, abstract open eye, containing within its center a vertical almond-shaped opening like a cat's half-dilated pupil. Behind this, a portion of the white, free floating, rectangular movie screen is visible against a black background. The edges surrounding the almond-shaped opening overlap at top and bottom, indicating that they are retractable, allowing the movie screen to be fully revealed or hidden. The black side walls and the white ceiling of the theater slope down toward this floor to ceiling black circle and are covered in black matte material on the sides that could also be used for the projection of images. These side walls were meant to create an experience of ever-expanding space, much like today's IMAX. Kiesler named his invention the screen-o-scope. The viewer looked forward at an eye looking back at him and then looked through it, to see the film projected on the screen on the other side. This design presented the viewer his eye as one end of an axis and the movie image as the other. It vividly illustrates how some images we can make ourselves as internal and imaginary, while others we can receive as externally projected back towards us. In both cases, our brains are always performing a complex integration of visual information in order to make sense of what we see. When we look at the open eye before the film begins, we are reminded that movies are first and foremost seen with our eyes.

The images or memoryscapes that at times occurred in front of my mind's eye during a migraine were similar in many aspects to their originals in the external world, much like frater-

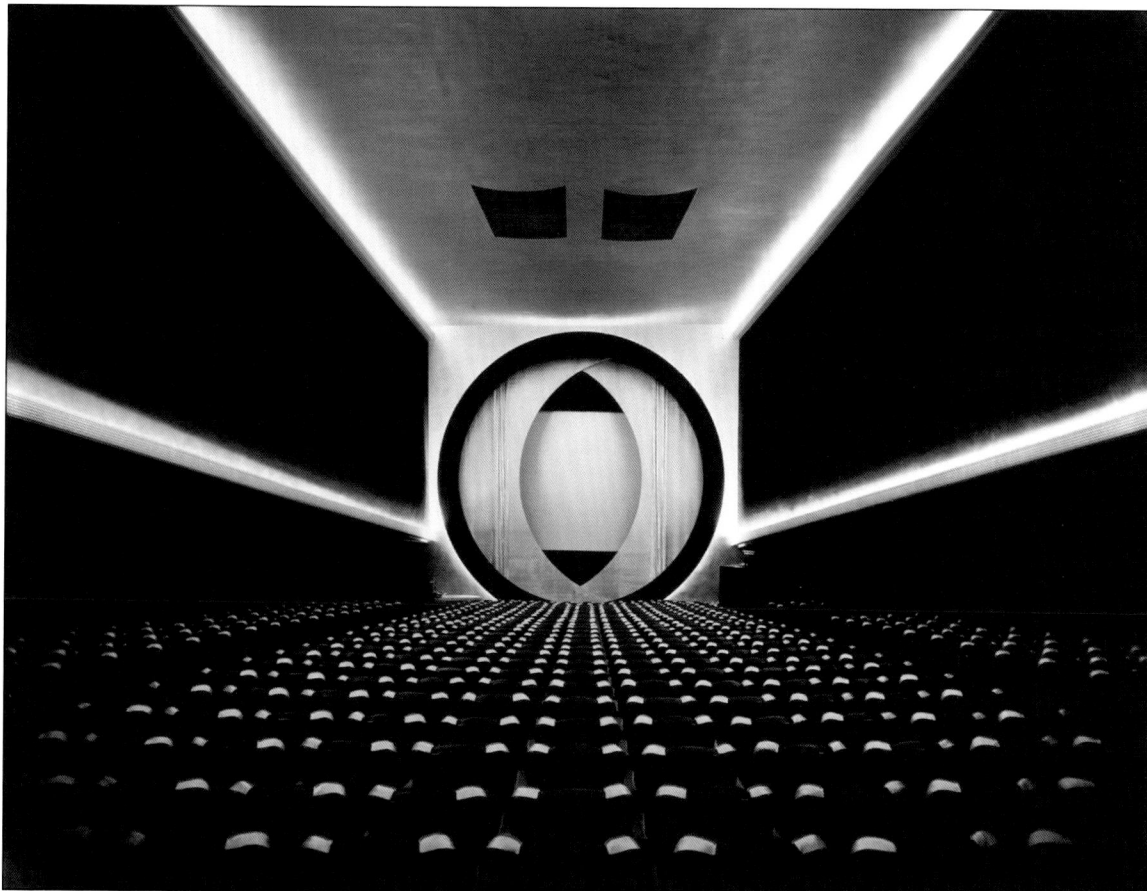

Friedrich Kiesler's Film Guild Cinema

nal but not identical twins. They had their own character that made them not quite of this world. These internal images first flashed spontaneously in front of my mind's eye, then achieved a certain objectification once I began to be able to recall them to mind. It was almost as if they were movie stills being projected back at me as made objects, ready to be rebuilt and manipulated. As I look at the eye and the screen in the Kiesler Cinema, I am reminded of the transit between the image of the original landscape in the external world that resides somewhere in my memory and its transformation via my imagination into a memoryscape.

Most neurological disruptions I experience that intrude on my field of vision are the result of migraine. They are not memoryscapes. Migraine disease has a centuries old history, and with that history come evolving definitions and treatments. One current working definition is that migraine is a collection of symptoms in response to abnormalities of neurochemicals within the brain, particularly affecting the part that processes pain. Once those responses get started, there's a multitude of downstream effects that involve nearly all the parts of the brain. This definition provides one explanation for the source of the myriad symptoms I experience during different phases of an attack. What actually causes this abnormal brain activity is still not well understood. Currently, much research on migraine disease centers on how neurons inside the brain misfire and set off a sequence of neurological events. It's thought that this is caused by genes that regulate the excitability of these neurons in the cerebral cortex in the brain stem. Greater excitation of the networks than normal has been recorded during migraines. These nerve signals then fail to regulate the effects of light and sound during a migraine. Migraine has no known cause but perhaps can have many triggers that trip an excitable nervous system. Loud sounds, flashing lights, alcohol, strong smells, cheese, chocolate, too little sleep, too much sleep, hormonal changes, stress, fluctuation in barometric pressure, or perhaps no triggers at all may be at work. It seems that the brain prone to migraine exists in a state of heightened awareness always with a low threshold of nervous activation that makes it ever ready to respond to the combination of stimuli that will trip the body's nervous system into a migraine. There are over one hundred and fifty types of migraines, each accompanied by a multitude of symptoms that occur at different times during the four phases of the migraine: prodrome, aura, attack, and post-drome.

I experienced my first migraine attack in October, 2003. The migraine worsened as the days progressed and became continuous: ebbing, flowing, and intensifying for many months but never subsiding. I sought help at the Jefferson Headache Center in Philadelphia where I became Dr. William Young's patient. He has been my doctor for the last nineteen years. My migraine was diagnosed as New Daily Persistent Headache, a sub-set of chronic migraine. It is a sudden headache that often accompanies the onset of a viral illness in a person who has had no previous migraines and is characterized by unremitting pain that is often resistant to treatment. In my case, eventually I did have migraine free days and even some months with very few migraines, but normally I have between ten to sixteen days a month with a headache. Though there is no one specific treatment for New Daily Persistent Headache, a range of medications are tried that are useful for chronic migraine, and some do prove effective. At times, the migraine seems to just burn itself out. Three-day outpatient infusions have been useful, as well as a longer five-day hospital stay. The prognosis is poor if the migraine does not resolve within the first three months. This has been my case. Even though I have tried to manage what I suspect to be my triggers, there seems to be no consistent pattern to my migraines other than a consistently prolonged rough period every year between August and October during which the headache is continuous and resistant. I have received excellent care from a team of nurses and from Dr. Young, who regularly guide me through a plan of treatment for these attacks when preventative and abortive medication are less effective.

One of a number of symptoms I regularly experience during a migraine, along with fatigue, mental confusion, poor balance, light and sound sensitivity, nausea and muscle pain, is the loss of orientation in space. The white smudges and flashing phosphenes that spread across my field of vision alter my perception of place dramatically. The visual assault takes the form of swarming particles that move in all directions, creating oddly shaped showers of fireworks and explosions of trailing, arc-shaped dissolving lights that form behind other opaque smudges that move at a slower rate across my vision. At other times, more compact and slower-moving expanding fortress-walled zig-zag patterns appear and slowly bloom. In more violent moments, bomb-like blinding, pulsing white lights originate low in my visual field and produce extended flickering. Sometimes these flashes and disruptions last for minutes, and at other times they last for hours.

Although terrifying, these phenomena are painless and silent. As they persist, I begin to lose my sense of orientation. Pain often follows. At times I become so disoriented I imagine I see myself as a small figure within the chaotic scene. Today, even twenty years later, when I experience this loss of orientation in space, this groundlessness, I begin to lose my sense of self, of who I am. I feel myself slip away from myself as the effects of the migraine eradicate the landscape in which I am anchored. It is as if I am being sucked into a featureless void that surrounds and envelops me as it moves forward through the shapeless darkness into the foreground of my vision. The edges of my body begin to feel as if they are blurring as I become more and more unstable. I feel like I am floundering in a rough sea illuminated by unsteady flashing lights. The displacement and fright accompanying these visual changes has left a deep imprint on me over the years as these episodes have become a part of my life. I have become accustomed to their visual brilliance but I never fail to be deeply disconcerted by them. To be oriented in space and time, to be assured of a continuous presence in space, no longer seems a given. The static quality of the memoryscapes, their reassuring stability, their provision of refuge within the swirling void, creates a solid landscape that offers me an antidote to chaos and dissolution, just as the static quality of the dioramas do.

In the early years of my migraine disease we had one goal: to eliminate the migraine. Dr. Young has been as unrelenting in the pursuit of this goal as he has been inventive in the search for effective medication. If there has been a migraine "warrior," a term popularly applied to people living with migraine disease, in my case, he has been the "warrior." He remains focused on ways to outsmart an enemy that is elusive and mutable. I have lost a lot that I have not regained: sound and light sensitivity have taken away moving images, music, much social interaction, filmmaking, and many good times with my husband and children. And yet, this ongoing loss has yielded new experiences.[1]

CHAPTER THREE

AT THE RANCH

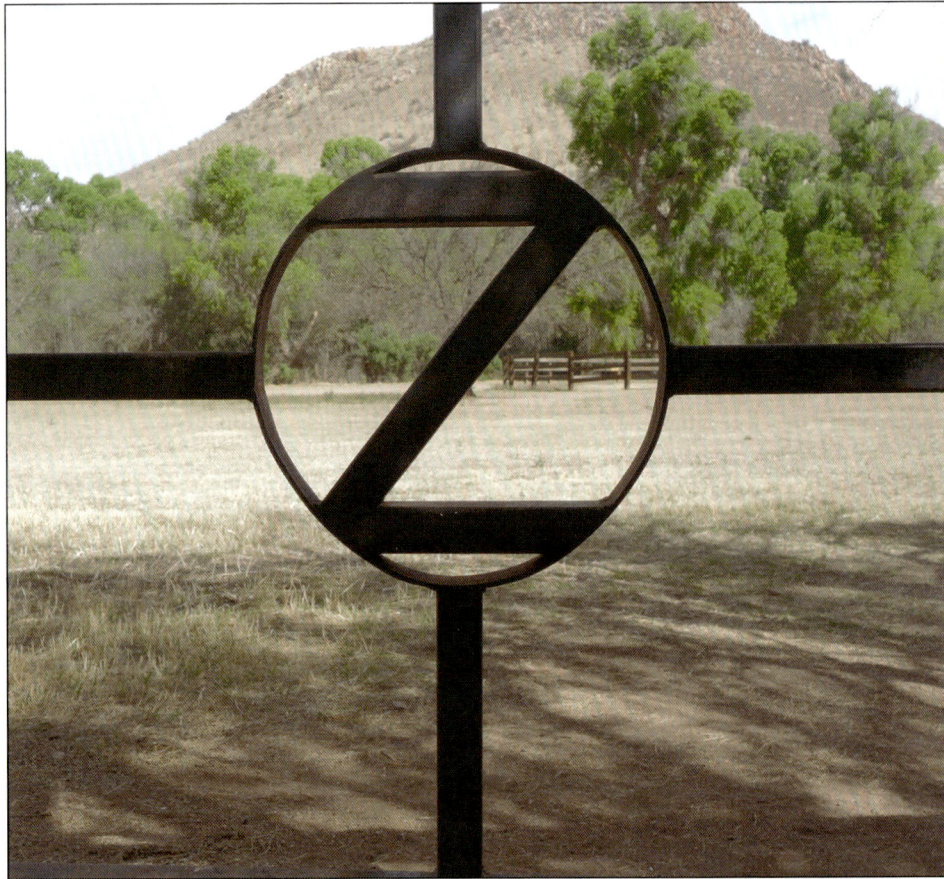

Gate detail

I awake not long after I have fallen asleep. The bedroom is cold tonight. It's late March in Chicago. Downstairs, all the suitcases are lined up by the front door, ready to be loaded into the taxis that will take us to Midway airport, a thirty-minute ride from our house near Lake Michigan on Chicago's South Side. The route over streets still littered with piles of dirty winter snow takes us due west on a wide boulevard lined with rows of two-story, squat, semi-detached houses constructed of gray Chicago brick. Their small front yards cushion them a bit from the noise of the busy street. My two sisters, brother, and I shiver together and watch the pools of florescent light from the street lights dissolve into each other. As a twelve-year-old in 1955, the trip ahead excites me. We will travel in a DC-6 that takes off on time at midnight and pitches itself above the vast lighted city, heads west towards Tucson, and touches down six hours later. I am bursting with anticipation and attentive to the new sights travel presents. At the airport, we children are pushed aside behind the luggage while our parents manage the tickets. Once inside the noisy airplane cabin, the mesmerizing tempo of the four grinding engines and the irregular, disorienting bursts of turbulence ensure we won't sleep.

The blackness outside the oval windows provides no answers to our questions about what lies below and beyond. I do know that this place toward which we are headed is special because we children have been included by our parents in their own incessant travels.

In an early brochure, Lee Zinsmeister, the owner of The Circle Z Ranch, insisted on calling his ranch a guest ranch, not a dude ranch. But Circle Z was in fact firmly rooted in the dude tradition that began when, after reading an article in a New York newspaper in 1883, Theodore Roosevelt headed west to hunt bison in the Dakota territory. He was perhaps the original dude, a sharp dresser, an educated, wealthy Easterner. In 1884 he returned west again, after the death of his wife and mother, to experience the restorative benefits of hunting and the cowboy life. Soon he owned two ranches, the Elkhorn and the Maltese Cross, and continued his friendship with his neighbors, the Eaton brothers, who were inviting other Easterners as non-paying guests to hunt and ride and experience life on a working cattle ranch, just as Roosevelt had when he arrived. Word spread quickly, and once the Eaton hospitality was extended to its financial limits, the dude ranch business was born as guests began paying for room and board.[1] These Easterners became known to Westerners as dudes because of the fancy cowboy outfits they wore and how they wished to imitate the ways of the locals who worked these ranches. Dudes were both mocked and coveted. Their welcome was assisted by a plunge in post–Civil War cattle prices that made this new way to monetize the land very attractive. Cattle, cowboys, horses, and the myth of the American West were Circle Z's birthright and the engine of its growth as a part of the new dude ranch tourist industry that flourished in the 1920s.

In the fall of 1926, the Zinsmeister family opened The Circle Z Guest Ranch in southeastern Arizona to twenty-four paying guests. Soon it expanded to accommodate seventy. Five miles south of Patagonia and fifteen miles north of Nogales on the Mexican border, the ranch initially spread over 5,000 acres, fanning out over the Sonoran landscape from the base of Sanford Butte, or Circle Z Mountain, on land that was originally homesteaded in 1867 by Denton Gregory Sanford. He ran a cattle operation until he sold off his cattle to acquire the 13,000 sheep he hoped would be more profitable. The Zinsmeister brothers, Lee and Carl, bought the failing Sanford spread in 1925. The old hacienda is still visible as a soft mound of adobe bricks on a low rise on the far side of the Sonoita Creek. Today, Circle Z owns more than 6,500 acres, many of which are conservation protected land.

In the twenties and early thirties, guests often arrived at Patagonia on the Southern Pacific Railroad or the New Mexico and Arizona Railroad in private railway cars that were shifted onto sidings to wait there to take them back east at the end of the season. These first guests were treated to a tableau of Western life created by Circle Z that consisted of morning and afternoon trail rides on the ranch's sturdy string of quarter horses, barbecues, rodeos, calf roping, polo matches, and cowboy entertainment. Ranch life remains essentially unchanged today, minus the polo matches. These activities nurtured a developing tradition that encouraged families to return again and again with their children and their children's children. Soon, returning guests considered the ranch a kind of second home, an unchanging one in which they felt an affectionate, enduring comfort and an emotional if not actual financial ownership. For nearly a hundred years daily routines at the ranch have remained the same: morning rides, optional afternoon rides, group meals, and a pre-dinner cocktail hour in the cantina. Modern incursions of phones, televisions, the internet and scheduled activities all have been held at bay.

After twenty years, the Zinsmeisters sold the ranch in 1946. During these early years Lucia Smith came to the ranch often, first as an eleven-year-old in 1936. She and her Midwestern Ohio family became devoted guests. Lucia began a life-long love of horses at the ranch. In 1976, she and her husband Preston Nash bought the ranch from Fred Fendig who had owned it since 1951. He, too, had acquired it after also having been a former guest. When he was near retirement, it was rumored that he was considering selling Circle Z to either a land development corporation or a tennis resort. The Nashs came to the ranch's rescue. It still is owned by the Nash family. Under Lucia's leadership all the founding traditions of the ranch were re-invigorated; its facilities refreshed, its remuda of horses expanded, new riding trails constructed, land steadily acquired, and many acres set aside for conservation. Today, Lucia's son, Rick, and daughter-in-law, Diana Nash, run the ranch with the same love of horses and devotion to the land.

At seventeen, George Lorta, born to a local family in nearby Lochiel on the Mexican border east of Nogales, came to the ranch to work as a wrangler at the corral. George continued to work at the ranch and matured; along with his responsibilities for the care of the horses and the dudes he began to lead on the morning rides. Today he and his wife Jennie, with the help of their grown children, work as a team with Diana and Rick Nash as resident managers of the ranch. Rick and Diana have not only strengthened Circle Z's cowboy ranching birthright but have gone further to re-affirm its deep local roots by incorporating the Lorta family into its tradition as resident managers.[2]

The special attachment guests feel for Circle Z resides as much in the specific events that take place there as it does in the spirit of the place. This atmosphere is the result of a unique blend of custom, history, geography, and continuing inhabitation on the land. Circle Z's guests are both returning pilgrims and creators of new memories that they come to make for themselves and with their children. My experiences over sixty-five years of visits to the ranch created a rich loam of memories out of which the migraine rescuing images I came to call memoryscapes emerged. My parents, Bill and Ruth Crawford, loved Circle Z; together they made one hundred and two visits to the ranch between 1951 and 1998, their last being when they were eighty-seven.

Until I was twelve, my only experience with the West had been through the occasional movie at the Jeffery and more frequently as the background for the weekly episodes of the Lone Ranger I watched on our small, recently-acquired television, encased in its bulky wooden cabinet sitting in one corner of our living room. The landscape shown in these episodes appeared mostly as black and white flashes that served as the backdrops to the racing cowboys, their snorting horses, and their show-stopping abilities to pull up their reins and come to an abrupt halt. These blurred images now appeared before my mind's eye during the long airplane ride. I became more and more excited to be leaving Chicago and more confused about exactly where we were going. I couldn't imagine how it would be possible for me to climb up upon a horse and move across the same countryside that the Lone Ranger and Tonto spent their days racing about in. All I knew was flat Chicago and the ocean that was Lake Michigan. I had seen no cowgirls. Of much more concern to me was how it was possible that my besuited businessman of a father could feel so confident about his abilities on horseback?

After a bumpy landing, we descend a steep metal staircase and leave behind all the darkness and enclosed, urban routines of the long Chicago winter to feel washed clean by the pale light of the southwestern dawn. I shed my heavy coat, then my sweater, and wish I could release myself from the scratching of my pleated wool skirt. Then, after the loading of the suitcases, our father takes the wheel of a rented station wagon, and we begin the journey south to Circle Z. He drives fast. I begin to notice the clusters of white crosses appearing at regular intervals along Route 82. On our left, a pale, pink glow spreads across the hills and slowly expands upward as dawn dissipates and the land around us comes into sharper focus. Bleary eyed and irritable from lack of sleep, I look out the back seat window at an unfolding vista of desert and distant mountains, unimaginable six hours earlier. Bathed in the early morning light, the Piñitos Mountains rise, shadowless now, enveloped in a soft purple haze, far, far ahead in another country called Mexico. The narrow two-lane highway rises and dips as we move deeper into the dry landscape where for the first time I see the widely spaced mesquite trees and ocotillo shrubs with thorny branches that shoot up and out like fireworks from a shared base. The earth is dusky brown and covered with gravel and rocks. The morning sky brightens and finally turns the clear deep blue that reminds me of those late fall days along Lake Michigan where that same intense color makes the water as blue as the Mediterranean.

We finally arrive in Patagonia, a small town full of dust and inactivity; it is unlike any town I have ever seen. It makes no sense to me. Running right through the middle of the main street is an abandoned railroad track on a strip so wide that the town appears almost to disperse on either side. The main highway goes straight through it on the west side of the tracks, yet the buildings on the other side that look so far away and disconnected seem to be of equal importance. From the descriptions of the transcontinental railroad in my school books I know that many Western towns were built around train tracks, but the width of this strip hints at something more than just a quick rail stop to water the engines. Patagonia's main attractions slide by: the Wagon Wheel Bar, the post office, a small grocery store, the silversmith's shop, the Museum of the Horse, a small hotel, along with several curio shops. A couple of dusty streets cross the tracks; off these, a few streets run parallel to the main highway. They are unpaved and lined with simple wood-frame houses, many unpainted, some with big side yards with room for horses, trailers, or a barn.

Patagonia once was a flourishing mining town. In 1891, R.R. Richardson began buying mines in the Santa Rita and Patagonia mountains and soon developed a portion of his ranch where it crossed the railroad at the Sonoita creek at the town that became Patagonia. Thousands of Mexican American and Latino workers came to the area around Patagonia in the years that followed to work alongside Anglos in the silver, lead, and gold ore mines which were sprinkled throughout the Patagonia Mountains to the south and southeast of town. The mountains surrounding Patagonia are still pitted with networks of thousands of underground tunnels in which the ore was mined and loaded onto the trains to be shipped out of the bustling center of Patagonia.

By 1955, when we arrived, Patagonia was a small town experiencing hard times and a declining population of under six hundred, hopeful that the tourism dude ranches would bring prosperity to the area. Today, a third wave of mining is gaining momentum. The Hermosa Mine, known as South 32, plans to exploit the old Harshaw mining area just outside Patagonia. Beneath the old sycamores may lie the largest undeveloped zinc deposit in the world. If the plan for a fifty-year underground mine proceeds, it will devastate the surrounding landscape south towards the border, changing the environment and biodiversity of the land in which Circle Z is set.[3]

We head out of town and begin the final five miles to the ranch. Here the landscape changes as the road begins to follow the course of the Sonoita creek. I look down at a messy sprawl of ancient, Freewood cottonwoods lining the banks of the creek. Their leaves catch the light and begin to flicker in the slight wind. The road dips and rises sharply as it snakes alongside this moving riparian oasis. And then suddenly we are there, at the arched iron gate in the middle of which hangs the large Circle Z emblem. I hear the new sound of tires moving across a cattle guard as we cross over onto the gravel drive and enter Circle Z. The bulky shape of Sanford Butte, or Circle Z Mountain, crowds down upon me. It is my first impression of this place.

The ranch was everything Chicago was not: warm, open, coppery brown and dry. Like two images plastered side by side in my child's mind, for many years Circle Z and Chicago retained this bipolar symmetry. Eventually, as I grew and visited the ranch more often, this rigid dichotomy disappeared. The ranch became untethered from Chicago as its distinctive atmosphere became lodged in my mind.

Uncle Fred owned the ranch when I was a child. He wasn't my real uncle and he didn't particularly care for children. I kept out of his way and he kept his distance. Fred and Dad were fraternity brothers at the University of Chicago and when Fred bought the ranch in 1951, Dad bought a small percentage of it as well. With the purchase of a Hereford bull named Majestic Domino they became partners in a failed cattle breeding business, a far cry from the Sanford days. On that first visit I stood in a group of dudes along the fence of the dusty corral and watched the family's C4 brand sizzle as it was thrust into the hides of the roped cows at my feet, all of which was made possible by the cowboy-wranglers who deftly handed the branding iron to my dad or Fred at just the right moment. This was the essence of the cowboy drama perpetuated at the ranch in those days, in part real and in part facilitated for the enjoyment of the guests. My Midwestern urban parents donned their bolo ties and cowboy boots and shirts with great ease. We all became proficient riders. For many years, with a grouchy expression, young George would lug Dad's heavy ornate saddle, made especially for him by Paul Showalter, a long time Patagonia cowboy and silver smith, out of the tack room and saddle up his horse while Dad stood by adjusting his spurs. George and Dad tolerated each other for a long time, each begrudging the other his territory and then, in their way, finally acknowledging each other's authority.

Above all, the ranch meant freedom from constraint. The physical world I was allowed to move unhindered in expanded exponentially at the ranch, and with this freedom from adult supervision I explored new worlds. I wandered up and down the creek alone in the afternoons and occasionally caught glimpses of a Great Blue Heron flying low over the water between the giant cottonwoods. At the end of the flats on the far side of the corral, I climbed into the heavy bales of hay stacked in towers and hid while I looked up at the cobalt blue sky. In the afternoons I filled the pockets of my jeans with mica-flecked rocks and peered into the undergrowth at small brilliantly colored birds. Later, I ventured up onto the abandoned railroad bed that ran for miles in either direction on the far side of the creek. Behind our rooms I walked down into the dry arroyo bed and followed it among the rocks and small boulders until it passed into the metal-lined tunnel under the highway where I listened to the thumping sound the cars made as they passed overhead. As I matured I became comfortable crossing the creek and climbing up to the low mesa to explore the site of the old Sanford adobe ruins. Then I would continue to climb upward on the horse trails which encircled the mountain.

I understood this open space to be the antithesis of the flat, linear, urban grid I grew up with. I was learning how to move about in such a space that had much in common with the openness of the habitat interiors in the three-dimensional New York dioramas I eventually became familiar with. On the morning horseback rides, I gave myself over to experiencing the expanding landscape with its receding horizons. Years later, as a myopic adult, the enforced monotony of the "slow ride" to which George often assigned me made me realize how much more I learned by experiencing the landscape at this painstakingly slow pace.

Throughout my childhood we mainly flew on a commercial airline from Chicago to Tucson but a number of times we flew directly to the nearby small "international" airport located near Nogales in a twin engine plane flown by my dad. Swooping down low to buzz the ranch, he often insisted I look at some particular thing I usually didn't quite make out. What this experience did do was teach me the landscape in a different way. Freed from the orientation of highways and horse trails on the ground, these low altitude aerial views knitted the landscape together as quilted segments of tilting sky, rolling grassland, distant mountains, and snaking creeks, all colluding to situate the ranch differently.

As adult, on many March mornings at the ranch I would open the wooden venetian blinds on the back window of my room in Casa Rosa and look out at a tool shed. It was a primitive rectangular structure made of semi-opaque corrugated panels of poly bicarbonate plastic sheeting. Yellowed by the sun, its undulating walls were pitted with scrapes and clumps of dirt. Pancho, the gardener, used it to store his tools and other supplies. Inside, bits of coiled wire, dirt-encrusted hoes, broken clay pots, rakes and spades littered the improvised shelves lining the walls. All this debris lay carelessly strewn about, creating a display that looked like some collector's beginning effort at classification. So many curious objects displayed within a big box reminded me of a cabinet of curiosity or curio cabinet, many of which were in fact room-sized displays. The intrinsic beauty of physical objects and their arrangement in glass cabinets remains an essential part of every museum experience and is at the heart of each diorama. Unlike a memoryscape, which is a mental image with its own somewhat flat yet interesting thingness to it, the tool shed was an actual free-standing three-dimensional object-filled display; a habitat for tools. Moving about inside, I felt the same calm reorientation in space that I did in the Lion Diorama. It became a boxed refuge within the larger refuge that was the ranch. In retrospect, I realize just how much of a fore-taste it was of my coming interest in dioramas. The shed's open door provided a fixed viewing point, just like the slanted glass window of the diorama.

The shed had more in store, though. A daily surprise awaited me. For a few minutes just before sunset in late March, the entire shed looked as if it burst into flame and was transformed from the inside out into a fiery, glowing box. Just at the exact minute the sun dipped behind the hills and entered the shed's narrow back window, this unassuming plastic structure flashed gold. Each night, I rushed to capture this moment before dinner with my camera. From its peak illumination, the light died quickly, so notably out of sync with the more gradual twilight fade of the surrounding landscape. The shed was oth-er-worldly then, magically transformed, far more beautiful than

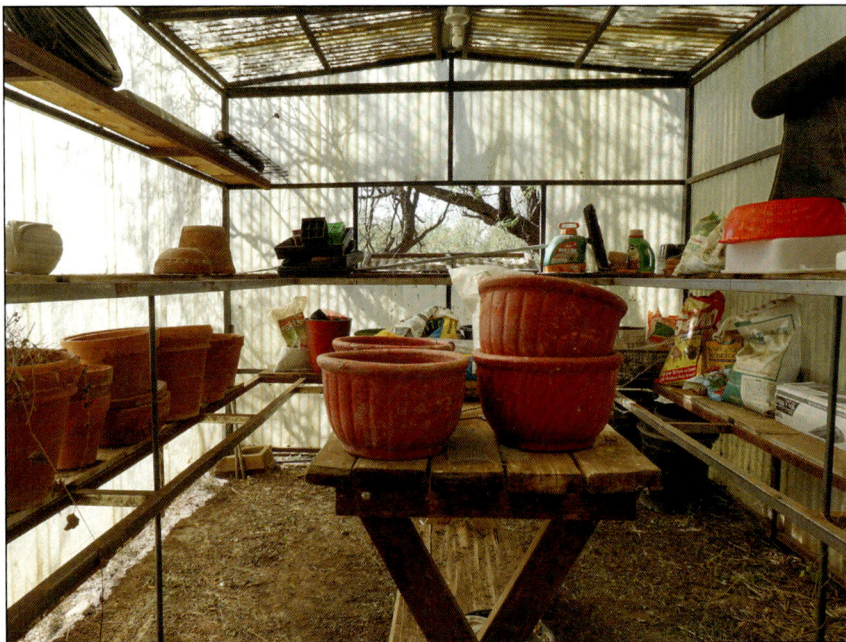

In the Tool Shed

Constance Dry

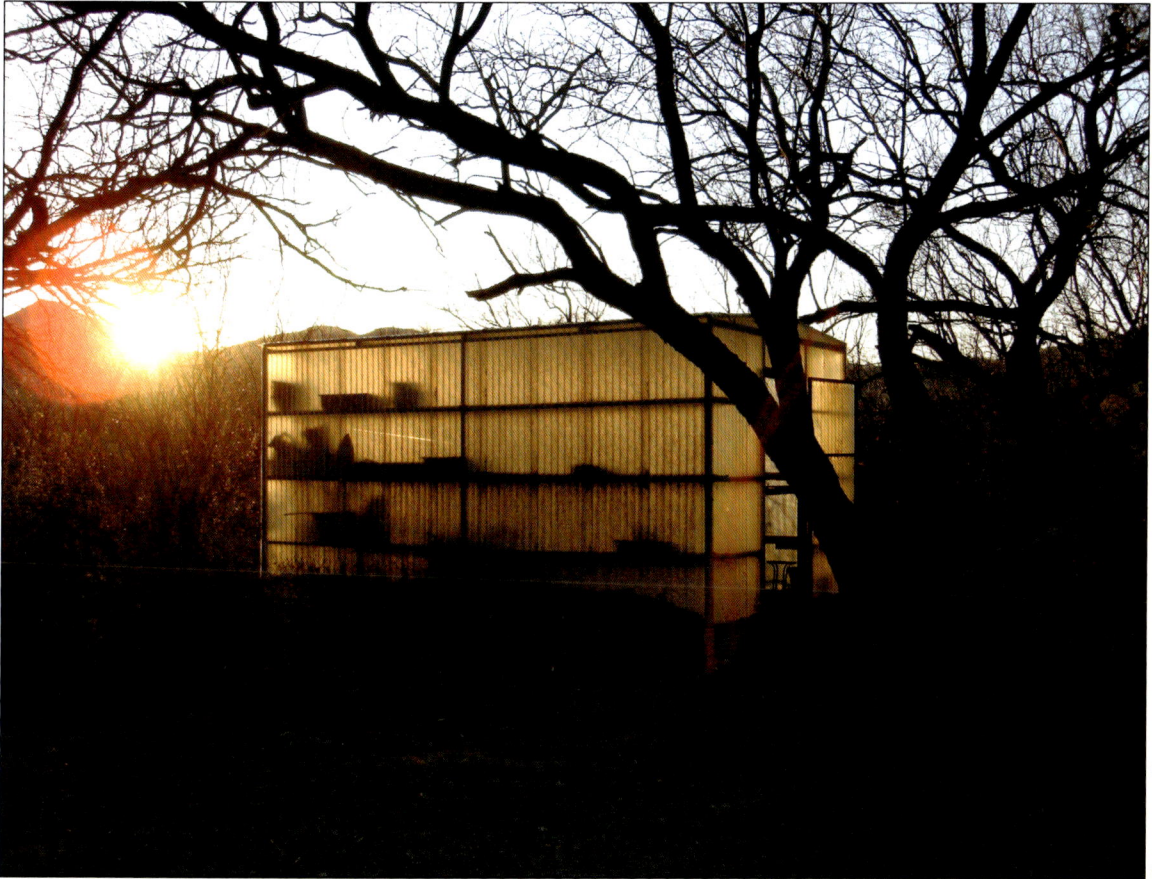

Tool Shed at Sunset

its muted natural surroundings. It was a common plastic structure made special by its relation to the surrounding landscape at the ranch.

Place is primarily defined by a particular location in space, but time also figures into how a locale became embedded in my memory. In addition to those in the shed, there were other special moments at the ranch during which time insistently stamped itself on the landscape. In these, I experienced place differently. Now I wonder if I should have been quite so amazed that Circle Z could have given birth to such objects of my mind's eye as the memoryscapes.

One warm day in March, 1988, I found myself leaning against the wooden corral fence to watch the horses run free toward their nighttime pasture. I looked down at the copper-colored gravel at my feet beginning to darken in the lengthening afternoon shadows. I glanced up to see that an edge of fluctuating green, formed by the spring leaves on the row of cottonwoods across the road, also deepened in the afternoon light. In the air over the gravel path between the fence and trees, thousands of dust particles hung motionless, suspended as if each were preserved in amber. At that moment, time stopped and all things material froze still, held in place, like the stopped moment in the stillness of a diorama. Present time, with its varying pace, halted and left me with a heightened awareness of the atmosphere of this place; the ranch and this landscape permeated me. This was not a spiritual feeling. It was more like a deepening understanding of my close connection to this locale.

In the years that followed, other similar time shifts occurred. Once, as the cook hurried across the lawn to ring the dinner bell, time present paused again in the day's last light. I saw the light fall on the black branches of the mesquite trees to create the same deep shadows on the neon-green grass lawn in front of the cantina. The sound of the clapper seemed to stop mid-strike and I saw each piece of gravel highlighted on the slopes of Circle Z Mountain in high definition. In that stopped moment, again, I absorbed Circle Z's accumulated presence on the land.

During a ride on another occasion, a nasty wind on a ridge behind Circle Z Mountain forced us to dismount for a rest. As I squatted on the ground, I squinted to see the sun disappear behind a fast-moving cloud. When I wiped the dust from my eyes time stopped again. In that momentary suspension of time's flow, the brush underfoot, the swooshing of the horses' tails, and the swaying of the ocotillo branches stilled as a momentary shadow fell. The land seemed to exhale in the shadow and re-affirm itself. And then time resumed. The blazing sun reappeared like a magnesium flash hitting a dormant camera plate.

Circle Z, as a place with its distinct geography, history, and aura, saturated my childhood and expanded its hold throughout my adulthood. Long before migraines and the emergence of the memoryscapes, its space and its feel set the stage for memoryscapes and my adult experiences with dioramas. The ranch continues to be a respite that provides sanctuary, year after year.[4]

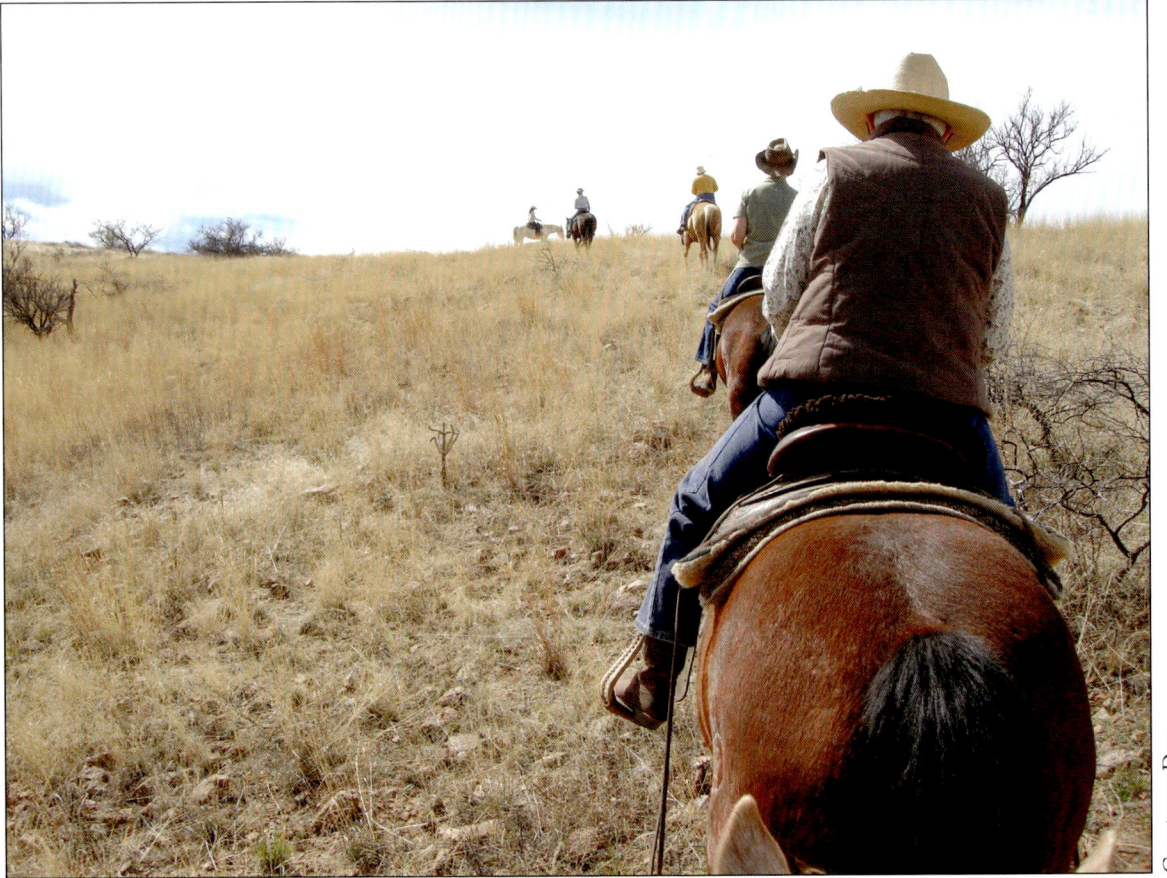

Morning Ride

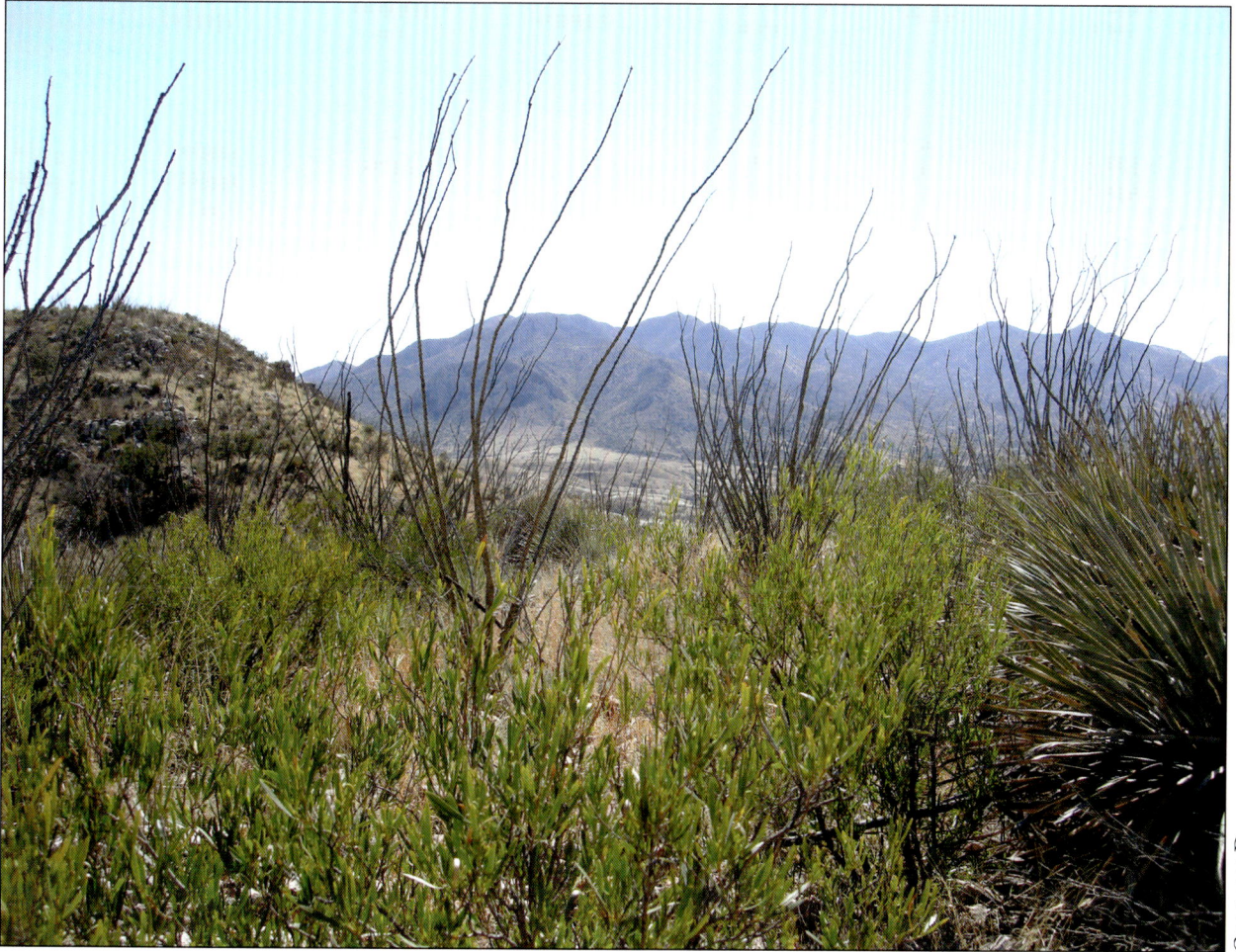

Ranch Landscape

Constance Dry

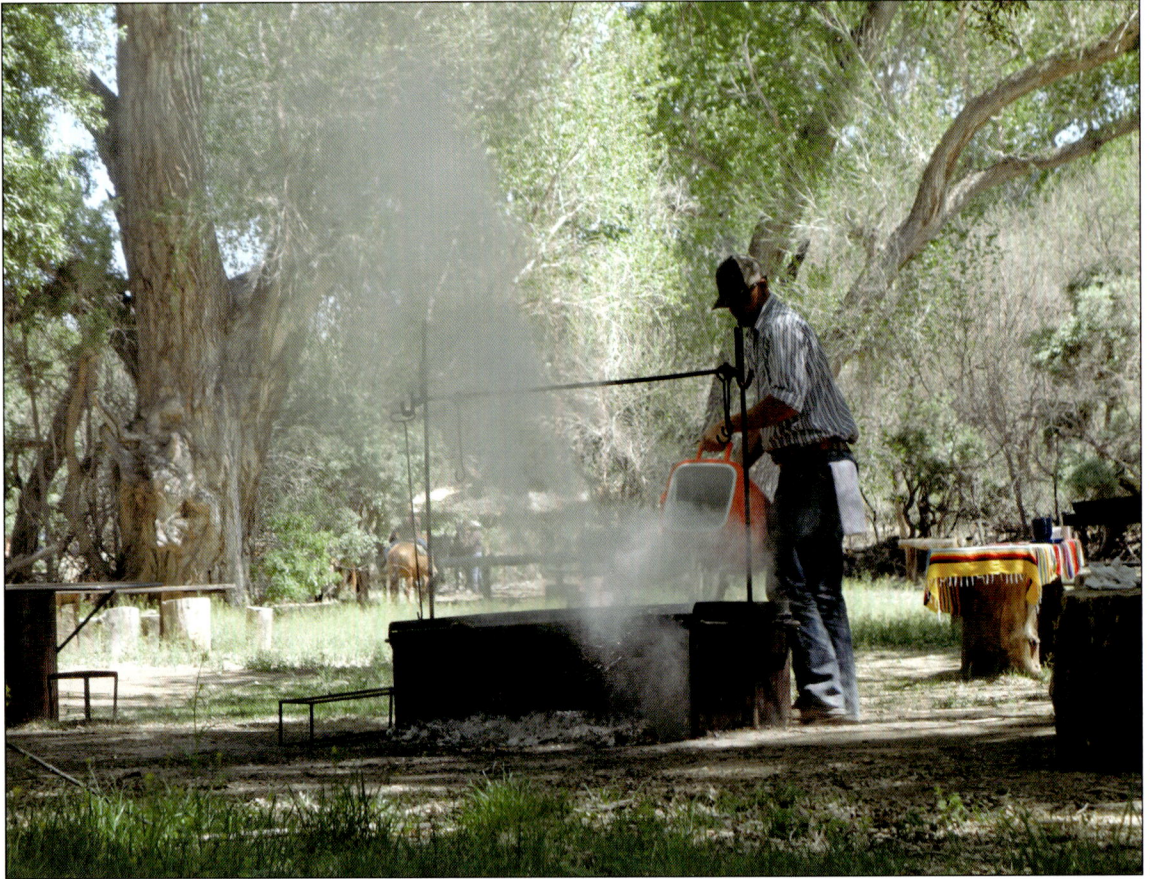

Barbecue Along the Creek

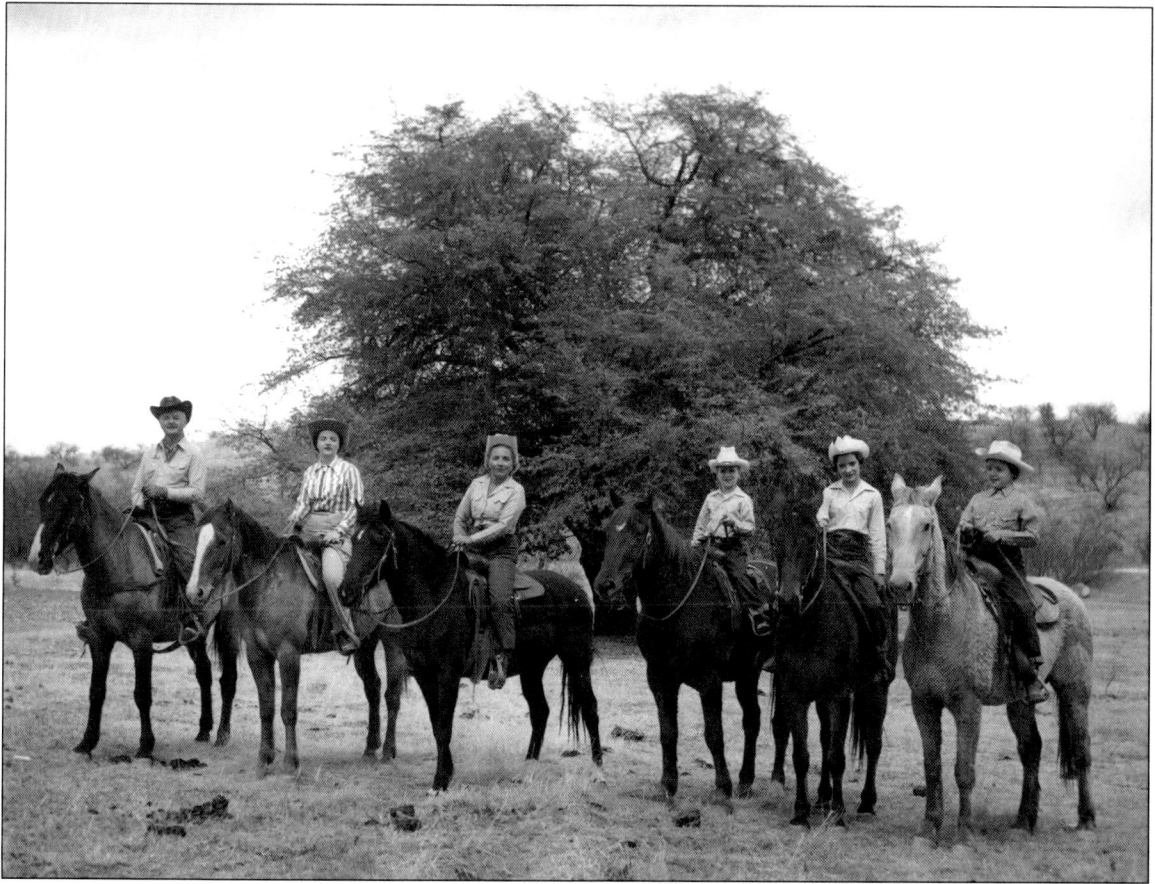

The Crawford Family in the 1950s

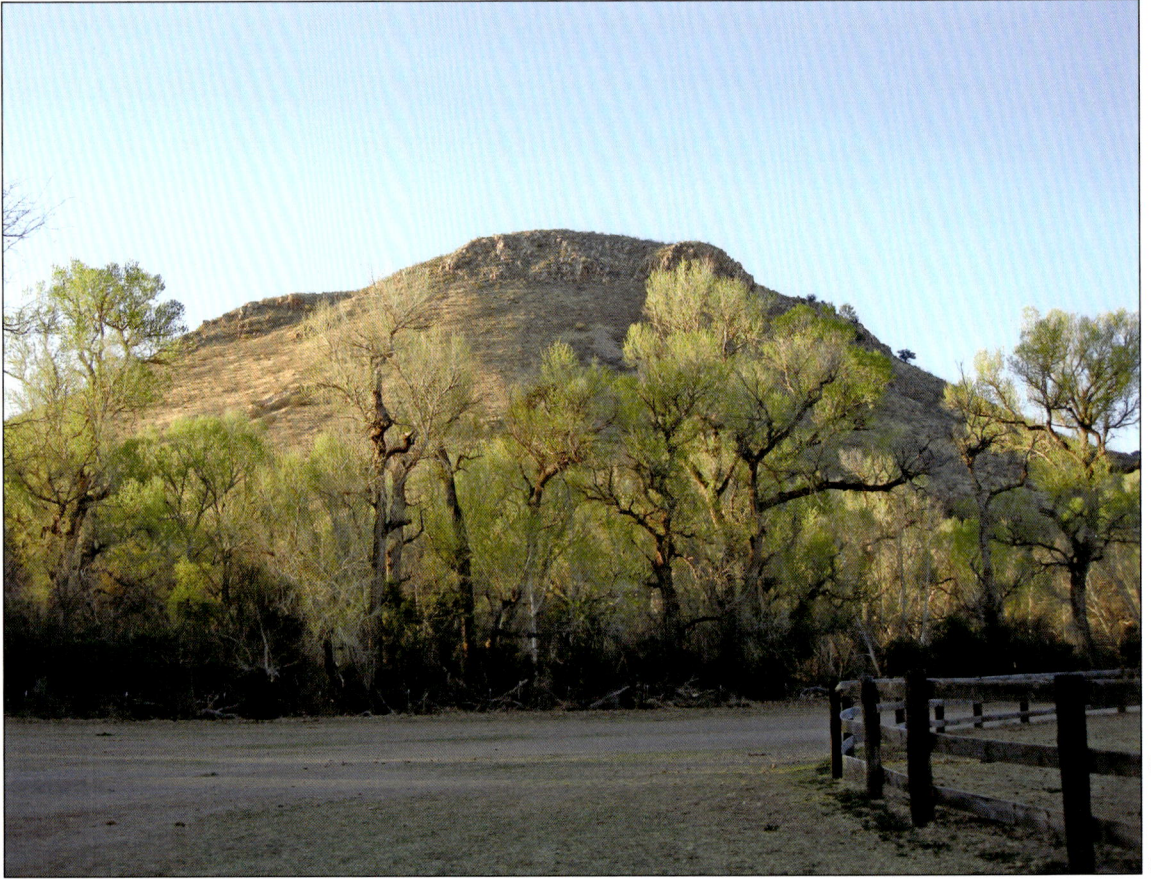

Sonoita Creek and Circle Z Mountain

CHAPTER FOUR

MEMORYSCAPES

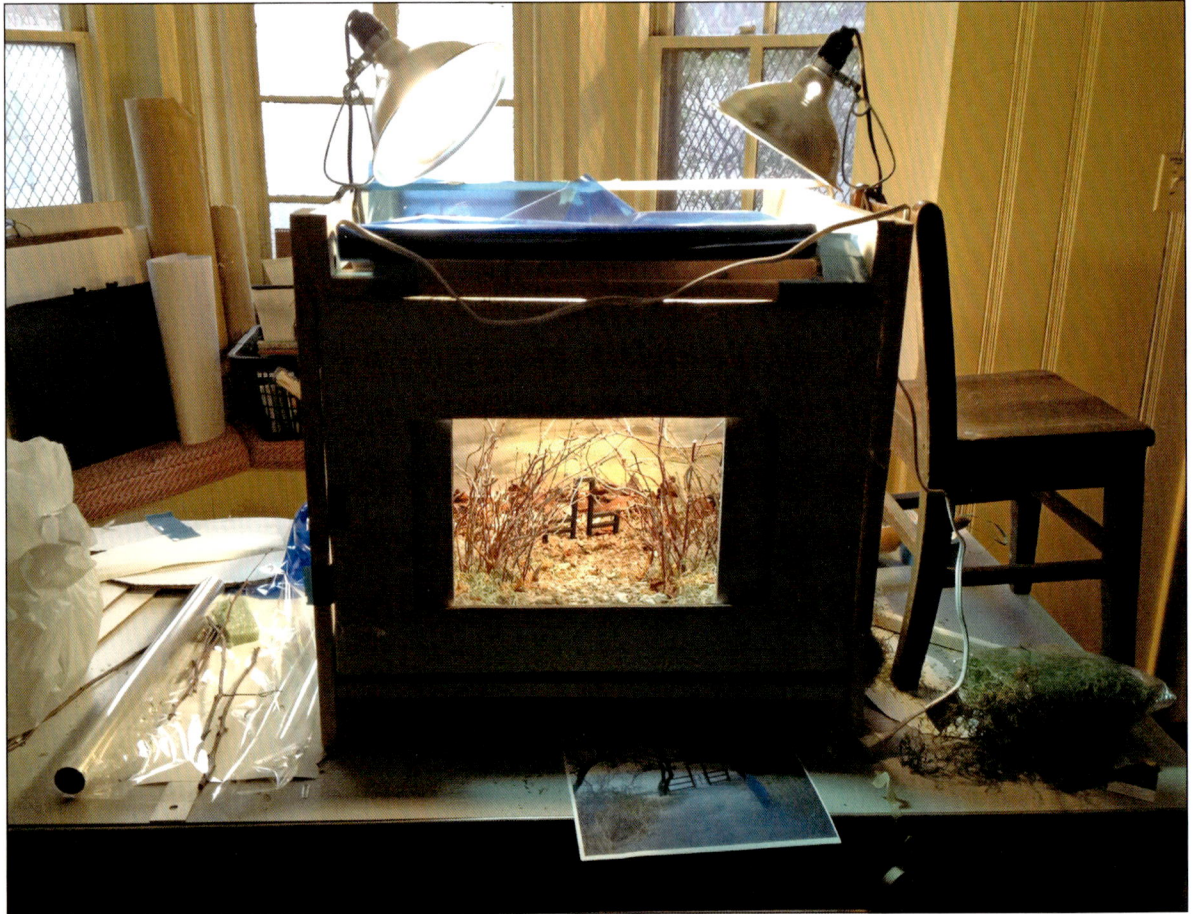

Gate Memoryscape, diorama

About five months after my migraines began, I started to carry a piece of frayed rope in my pocket. By then, my headaches were almost continuous. On this rope I tied a series of randomly spaced knots to mark the occurrence of migraine attacks. Fingering these knots reminded me of the unpredictable nature of my intractable migraines: smooth times, rough times, no consistent pattern. At first these knots signified the headaches themselves, but soon their meaning shifted and they began to mark my use of a growing inventory of memoryscapes that appeared to me during the initial period of daily migraines between January and September of 2004, a time when medication offered me little relief.

Although each image originally appeared spontaneously, in time I was able to call up at will these visual objects to my mind's eye during a migraine. Like the knots on the rope, they were way stations. By first viewing these memoryscapes and then holding them before me, I found relief from the tumultuous spatial and neurological landscape created by my brain during migraines. Through these images, I gained access to the grounded places of the world they presented that then became reliable places of refuge. The actual landscapes from which they originated were familiar to me at Circle Z. Therapeutic and beautiful, once I entered the pictorial space of the memory-scapes, each experience I had within was new.

How did they come about? As I lay enveloped in pain one morning, I saw something quickly appear in the darkness before my closed eyes. In that instant, a tableau of horses arrayed beneath an immense blue sky appeared in a rapid visual flash. The image looked like a colored film frame, slide-like, almost transparent, in sharp focus, dense with detail. The group of horses milled about in the outer corral at Circle Z. Flaring up for that fraction of a second, this image eradicated the disorienting blackness and bursts of light overwhelming me. I lay mesmerized in my tangled bed sheets in my darkened bedroom at midday. It was early February, 2004, and even though I was still besieged by continuous daily pain, I was fascinated.

This group of sturdy trail horses rested together under the morning sun. They distributed themselves across the lower third of the image. They were in sharp focus, and so looked real and yet didn't. Above, a translucent blue sky filled the remainder of the treeless image. The sun is bright; the morning cloudless. The horses either stand or lie resting on their sides. All is quiet. No dogs bark, no humans converse, no birds sing. An occasional truck with a diesel engine, or a jet's engine overhead, may echo faintly in the distance. Some horses seem to have recently finished rolling in the caked, dusty earth. Others stand, heads and necks extended downward to nuzzle bits of hay and grass. I sense these horses are the ones who have been left

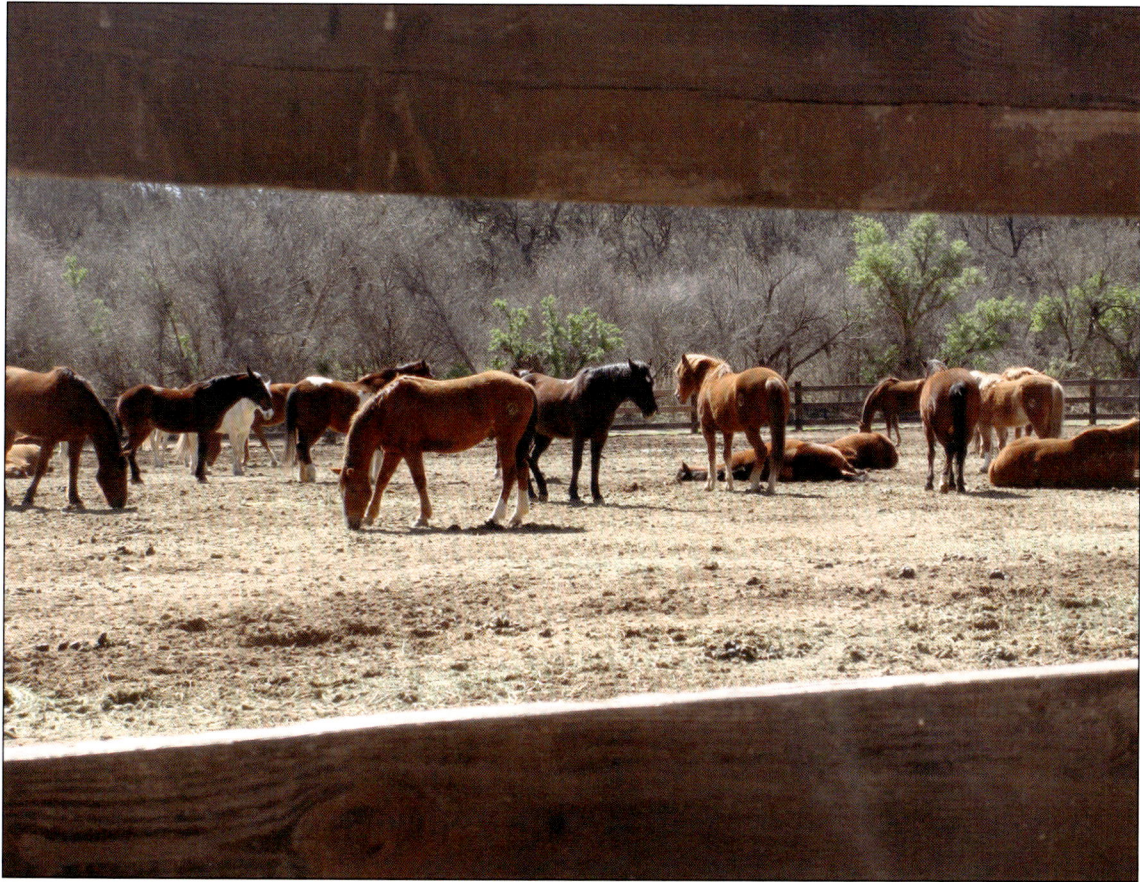

Horses in Corral, photograph

behind, not having been saddled up for the morning ride, and therefore seem to enjoy the quiet while waiting until the others return at noontime, when they will all be released together to run free towards the evening pasture. The morning's warmth, the horses' ease, the shower of bright, shadow-free light combine with the stillness to produce an aura of contentment that saturates the scene and washes away the neurological disruption. The intense cloudless blue sky pushes down onto this scene, directly falling upon the bodies of the horses.

The images of the mini-dioramas that follow are my attempts to make three-dimensional versions of what flashed before my mind's eye.

The unbidden image of the horses originates neither from a dream, nor a hallucination, nor out of a specific remembered event. It is at once detailed yet somewhat abstracted, comfortable to me in its familiarity. In my pain I try hard to hold it before my mind's eye. I look into the space created within the gently shifting group of horses and begin to move toward them and visually enter the shelter they create inside their loose grouping. There, I sense, I will find refuge. Maybe then I can begin to re-orient myself in space and rest and look up into the blanketing warmth of the sun. But before any of this occurs, the image abruptly disappears. The pain intensifies. The image's beauty lingers for a moment as an afterimage, hovering like a blurry imprint. I wonder if the corral and the horses will return. What was this? Where did this familiar yet hyper-real image come from, so unattached to any recollection, yet so evocative and familiar?

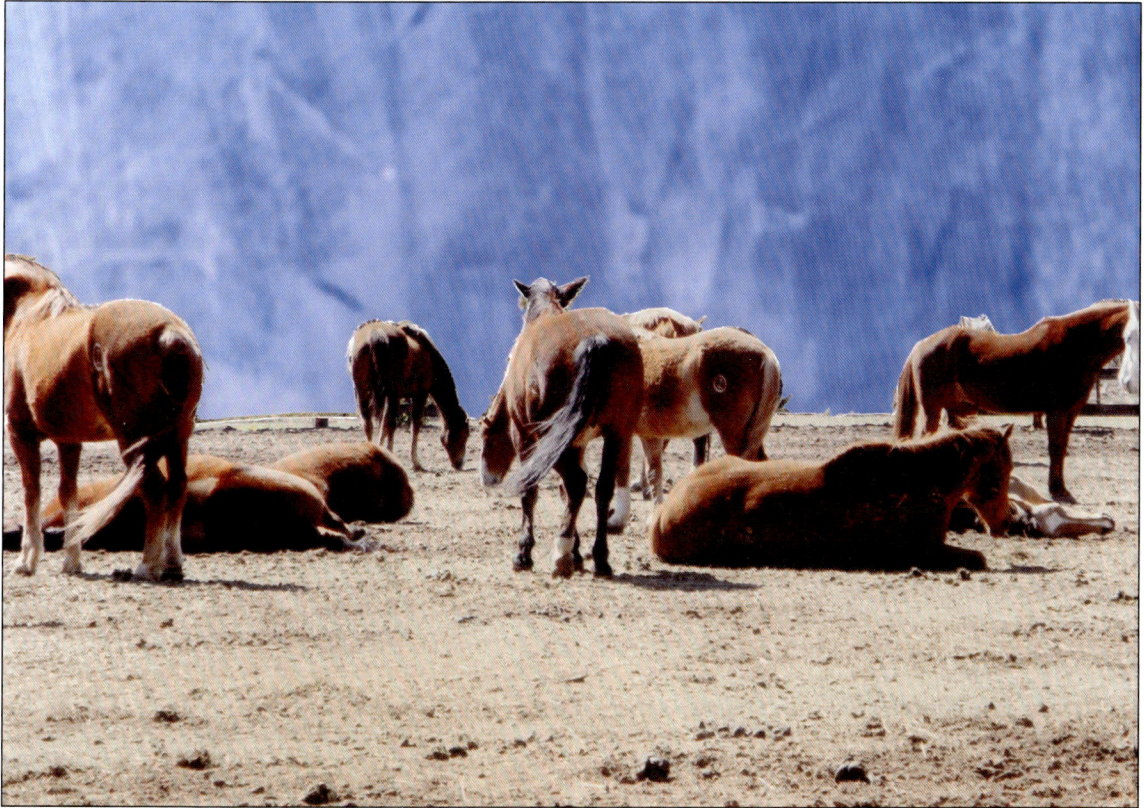

Corral Memoryscape, diorama

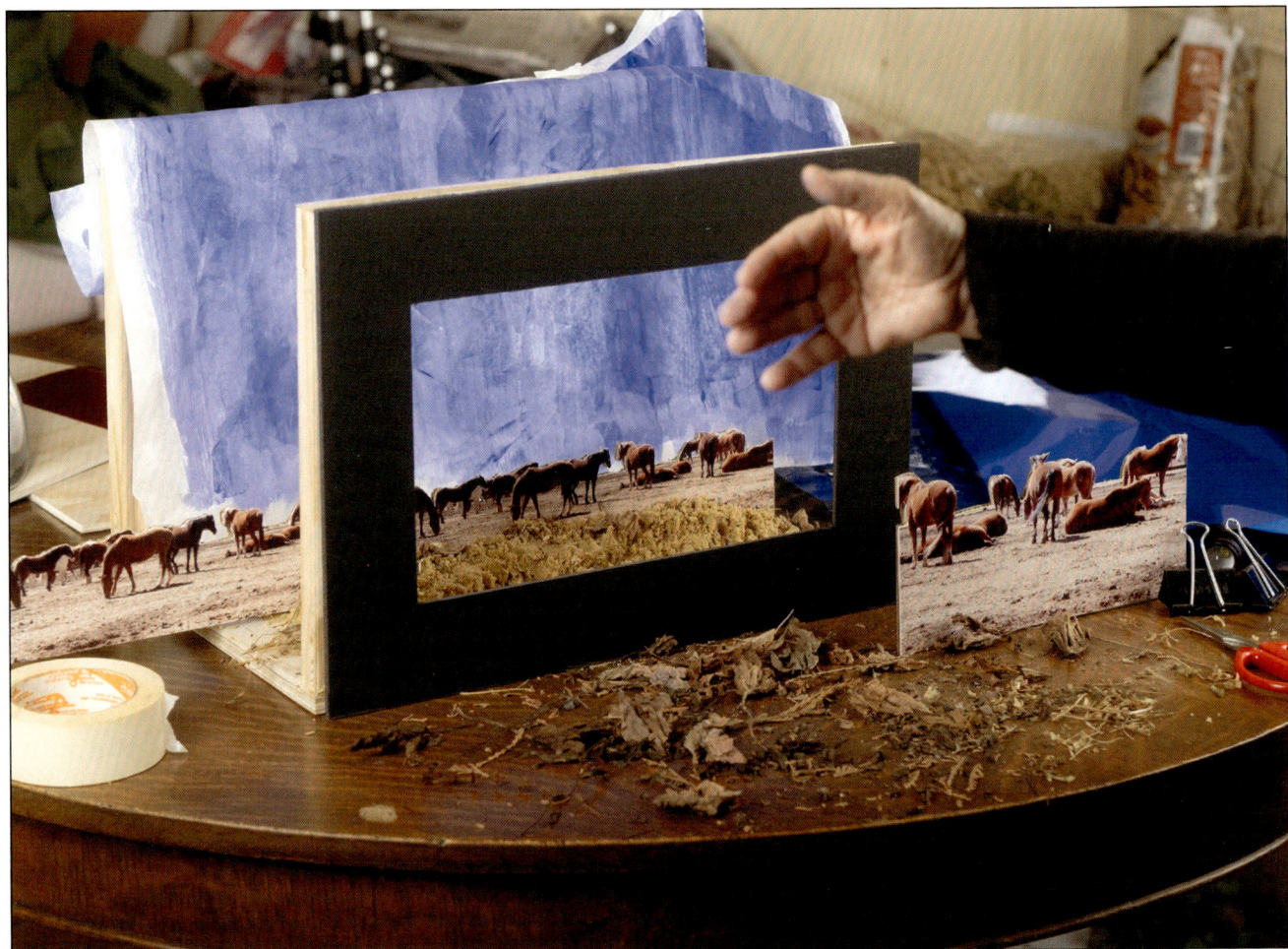

Corral Memoryscape, diorama

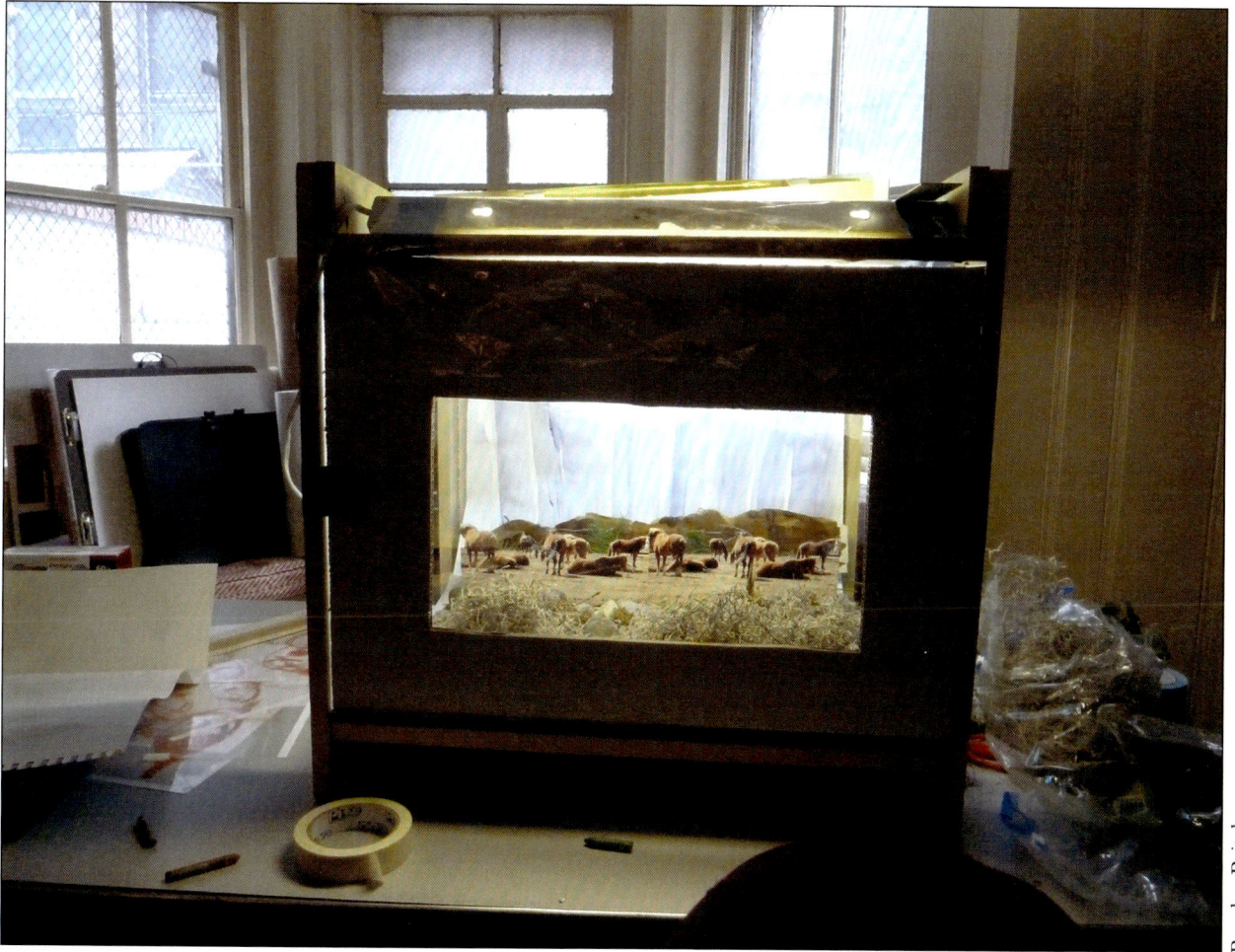

Corral Memoryscape, diorama

In the days following the Corral Memoryscape's first appearance, my migraine continues without cessation and I struggle to cope with the incapacitating pain. I wonder about this flickering mental image. I don't expect it will re-appear, but then, to my surprise, in a couple of weeks it does. As before, it arrives unbidden. Again, I see the same vivid scene of horses in a corral. When I view it, I begin to feel myself again grounded in space and place and the pain subsides. During the following weeks, I am surprised to see the image return more and more frequently. Each time, my desire and my ability to hold it in my mind's eye increases. By concentrating hard while it is in view, I meticulously begin to stabilize it. I hold the image as long as I can and then, in an attempt to keep it present, I begin to reconstruct it piece by piece from the ground up, holding each piece in place in my mind as I go. When all the pieces fit seamlessly together and the image is steady enough so that I feel sure of its solidity, I look at the whole memoryscape, confident that I can visually enter it. Like a jigsaw puzzle, each piece is securely locked into the adjoining pieces. I am not plastering over the neurological disruptions, I am replacing them. After much practice, I am able to recall the image at will and hold it there in front of my mind's eye. I hold the image together by this continual rebuilding. This effort diverts my brain from pain. Then I can reorient myself in space.

Once inside the enclosed space formed by the horses, I rest amongst them. My thoughts drift toward memories of childhood, of sitting on the cement driveway where I played endless games of jacks with my sister during the hot Chicago summer long ago. I throw them out again and again on the warm pavement. And then I remember the feel of my thumb and forefinger prying off the round metal sprinkler cap embedded in the lawn and the release of warm water in a fanning spray. Other images begin to surface. Some re-appear and shine brightly before me while others are vague and insubstantial. I am one step beyond the anchoring corral, now.

During severe migraines, I also call up the Patagonia Mountains Memoryscape. It, too, brings to mind thoughts of the ranch and its reassuring presence. Awake at night the pain begins in my face and courses all the way down the left side of my body. In search of refuge, I look into the memoryscape that begins across the road from the entrance gate to Circle Z and extends beyond to the Patagonia Mountains. They are arrayed across my vision as a string of distant, gently sloping hills and mountain ridges. The last rays of the setting sun break across their southwestern slopes and turn them a fiery copper. This elongated image is slightly curved at the edges and framed by a thin black line. Emerging night, pale and violet, rises off the uneven horizon and deepens to aquamarine and cobalt higher up in the darkening sky. The view is to the east, away from the sun. As in the Corral Memoryscape, an immense, clear sky fills three quarters of the image. At its base in the foreground, across the road, the low-lying scrub, cactus, and mesquite covering the rocky hillside has already darkened. On the rise above it, the bare branches of mesquite trees entwine to create an interlocking scrim that occupies all the midsection of the image. This curtain of interlacing black branches balloons up out of proportion, appearing larger than what is actually seen at the site. The Patagonia Mountains look as if they rise up directly behind the trees, rather than in the far distance. The black branches grow incandescent in the rose light of the fading sun. The long, low, last rays of light penetrate this lacy screen and illuminate its interior space. Inside it glows, just like the interior of the tool shed at sunset. This large shape, elongated like a glow worm cocooned in mesquite branches, sits humped on the ground, asserting its importance as a place of refuge. The heavens, with the evening star just visible, rise up above this scene like an inked scroll unrolled to reveal more and more of the emerging hues in the night sky. They are as vast as the migraine's black, disorienting, tumultuous void, yet here they calm rather than frighten.

Once the whole image settles in front of my mind's eye, I move toward the puffed up, oblong shelter. The pain takes notice. I slip into it on one side, through the scrim of mesquite branches. Inside, I immediately feel the comfort the edges provide as they enclose the space around me. Calmer now, I slowly begin to reorient myself in space. The migraine's disconcerting void fades and now I can stand steady and upright in the center of this shelter. After a few moments I tilt my head up to peek through the ceiling of branches to the clear sky and

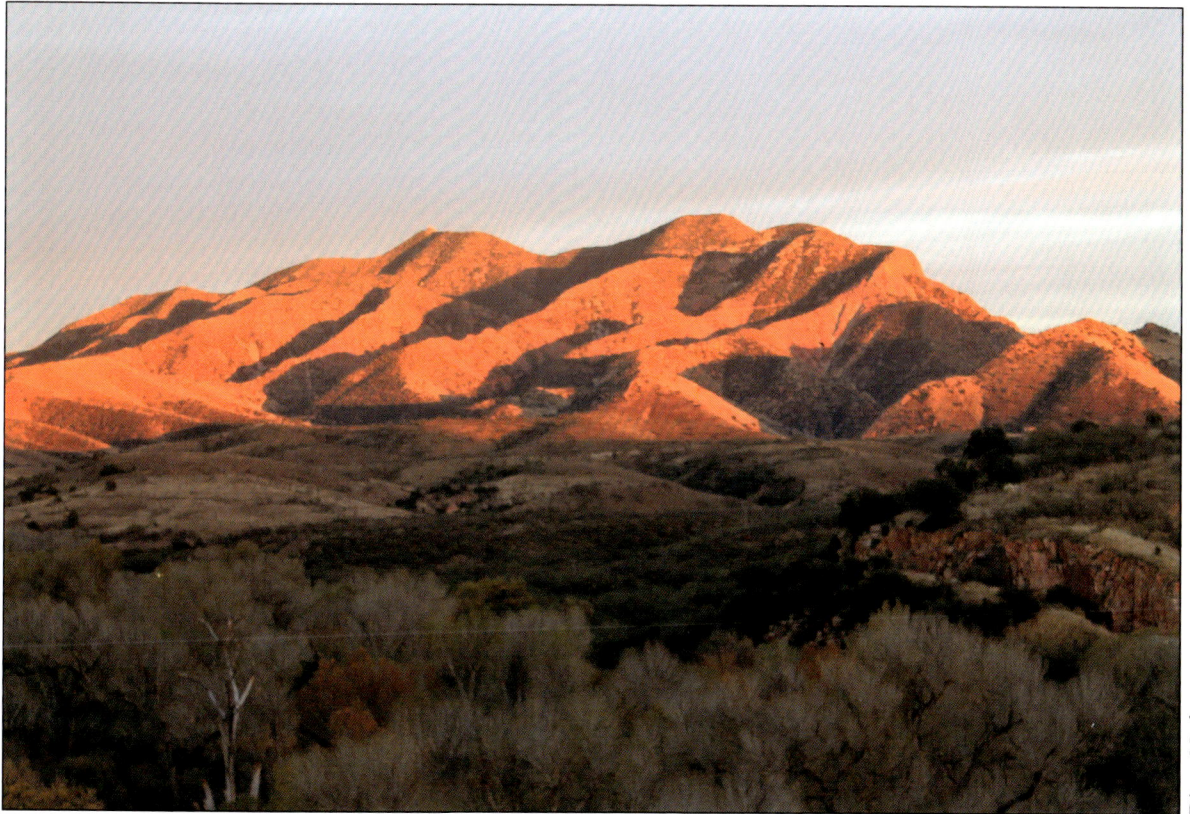

Patagonia Mountains, photograph

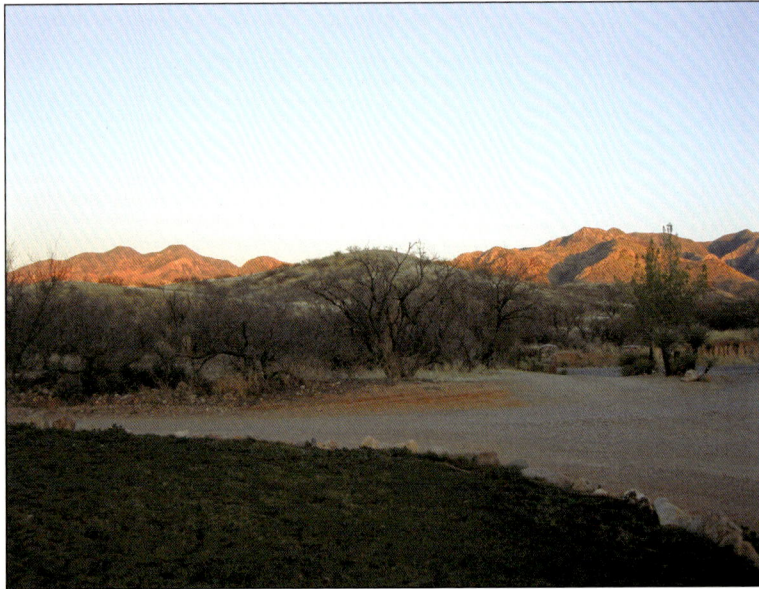

Constance Dry

Patagonia Mountains: photograph (above) and diorama (below)

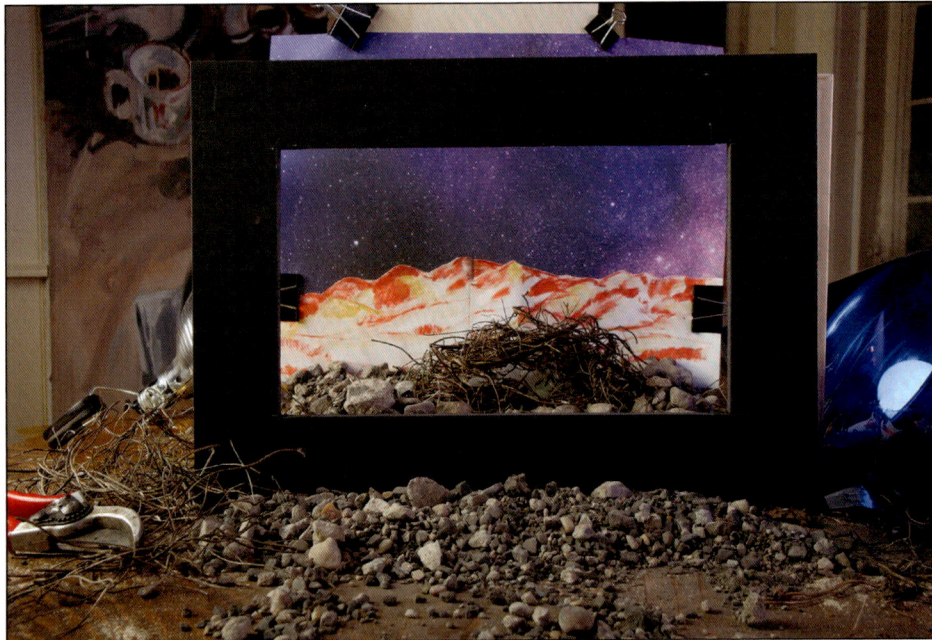

Justin Audet

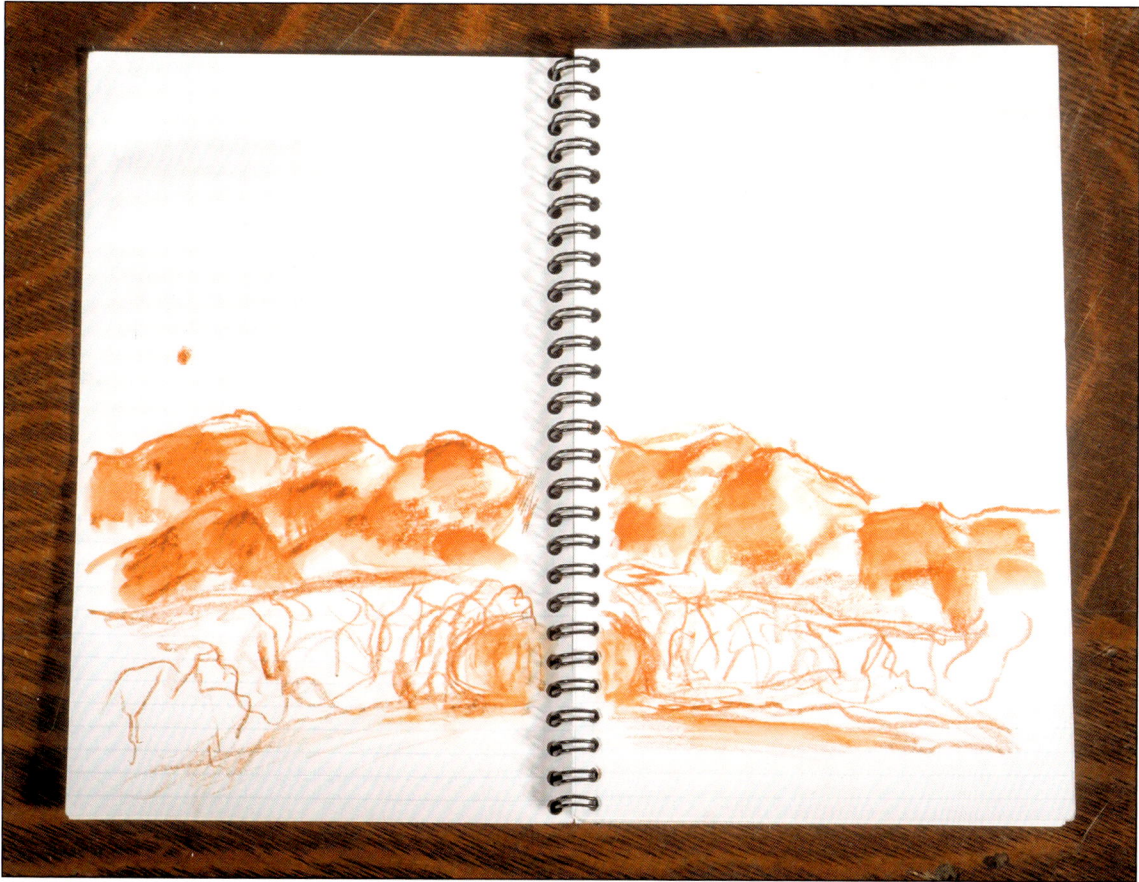

Sketch of Patagonia Mountains Memoryscape

the slow changing colors in the emergent night. I relax even more as the world the migraine creates stops swirling and the lights stop flashing. The sun is not visible, only the imprint of its last rays across the slopes indicates its rapid transit across the immense sky. The changing light attracts me. The violet sky darkens and deepens, drawing my gaze slowly up toward the heavens. Upwards and upwards I look, until I fully forget my pain as I immerse myself in the unfolding drama of nightfall. Now I perceive myself to be a small speck in this infinite but stable universe. Within this refuge I am steadied and reassured.

These mountains resemble the real mountains that begin south and east of Patagonia and run alongside Route 82 towards Nogales. At Circle Z Ranch they provide relief from the imposing presence of Circle Z Mountain by opening a view outward to the east that encompasses a more distant horizon. The oblong protected space formed by the mesquite branches that I see within the memoryscape is an exaggeration of a low rise on the other side of Route 82 that in reality is covered only by a thin sprinkling of scrub.

Though they are not exactly replicas, both the Corral and the Patagonia Mountains Memoryscapes are close enough to their earthly originals that their actual sites were easy to locate at the ranch. I often passed these sites during the day, yet never fixed them in memory as static stopping off points in my journeys; they were registered as bits, if at all, in the wider view, unnoticed in the overall fabric of the place through which I was moving. Both of these memoryscapes invented their own place. They contained faithfully rendered details of the original landscape, but they were changed enough that they became approachable in visually original ways.

But what were these two images, these memoryscapes of corral and mountain, that had such power to interrupt and transform? Each flash was an artifact of visual perception, both an image before my eyes and a seeming material object, made to be manipulated. They were both flat at first glance and then three-dimensional when entered. Perceptual objects, neither photographic nor painterly, that looked like hyper-real portions of a taken-for-granted landscape. Each shared with the other memoryscapes the same quality of intense, clear light, a level entry area, an indeterminate middle ground or deeper space, and a farther off, celestial exit point, all painterly conventions. These familiar visual bits, the raw material of the memoryscapes, must have existed somewhere deep in my memory, waiting on the sidelines of consciousness, like empty vessels, ready to surface when needed as life-like perceptual objects I could inhabit. Free of human beings, they were neither desolate nor alienating. Within them my inner unafflicted self, once stabilized, could act in imaginative ways. Diverted from pain, I moved away from it.

The Gate Memoryscape presented a slightly different perceptual experience. It evoked the other gate, the main gate at the entrance to the ranch, which was different in importance and construction. This one was smaller, set down low at the base of a sloping, dirt foot path that led to the corral. At the bottom half of this gate, in its center, a round circle with the letter z inside hung within a finely wrought square iron frame, similar in design to the one hanging from the main gate. A wooden structure supported this gate and focused my attention on the elegant, black shape of the letter z. Above it, wooden crossbeams created the outline of an outsized door, twice as tall as the open fencing, three boards high, that supported it on both sides. This structure with its latched gate separated the borderless path from a field beyond. Viewed from the top of the path, the gate and fence appear to float unanchored; other than a few strands of almost invisible barbed wire, I can't see any supporting extension of the fence on either side of the gate. In the foreground, a few wide, shallow steps cut into the path to ease the descent to the gate. On one side, the steep hillside is covered with grasses and mesquite trees whose overhanging branches shade the path. The bare field beyond is flooded with hazy light. In this field the soft shape of an old riding ring encircles the tree at its center and makes a faint impression in the distance. The entire memoryscape, unlike the site from which it is derived, is suffused with a blueish haze created by the overhanging mesquite branches that rise up in the foreground and spread across the top of the image. It is difficult to reconstruct this memoryscape in my mind's eye because the soft grays, blues, and beiges soften the sharp edges necessary for an easy jigsaw-puzzle-like construction. Unlike the others, there is no possible sheltered

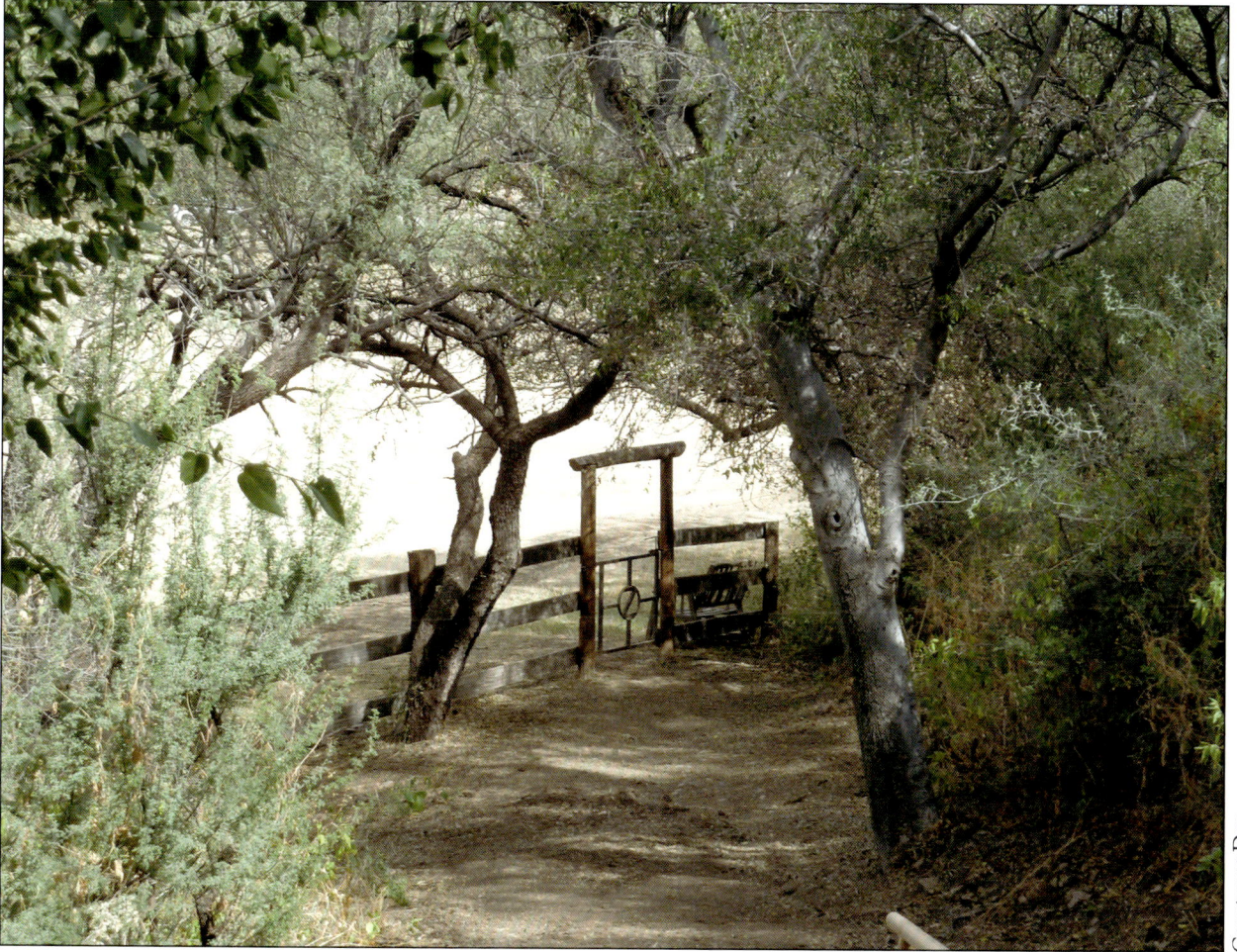

The Gate, photograph

Constance Dry

interior space within the Gate image to draw my eye forward. The circular path of the old riding ring is too vague to outline a place of refuge. Here, the dominant impression is of peaceful, safe transit across a boundary bisecting a muted, shadowless scene. The Circle Z emblem anchors the space and divides it in two. The field on the other side of the gate blurs into a softened, horizonless vista.

In contrast, both the Patagonia Mountains Memoryscape and the Corral Memoryscape look up to the sky, which appears as a vast nonthreatening open space that counteracts the disorienting void. From the shelter among the branches in the Patagonia Mountains Memoryscape I look up safely at the fast-moving daily transit of the setting sun; within the shelter provided by the resting horses in the Corral Memoryscape, the unmoving midday sun shines directly down, enveloping me in its stabilizing warmth. The Gate differs because it suggests unimpeded earthbound movement from one state to another. Gentle on the eye, it is a potent emblem of the possibility of a calm journey or the persistence of smooth untroubled times.

By November of 2004, I had returned to Circle Z for my sixteenth visit. A year had passed since the onset of migraine disease, when I had begun to regularly call up the memoryscapes. Their dependable reality as visual objects strengthened over time. On that visit back to the ranch I tried some experiments with my camera to see if the actual sites of the memoryscapes would match up with my mental images of them. I wondered why these memory bits originated in such unre-

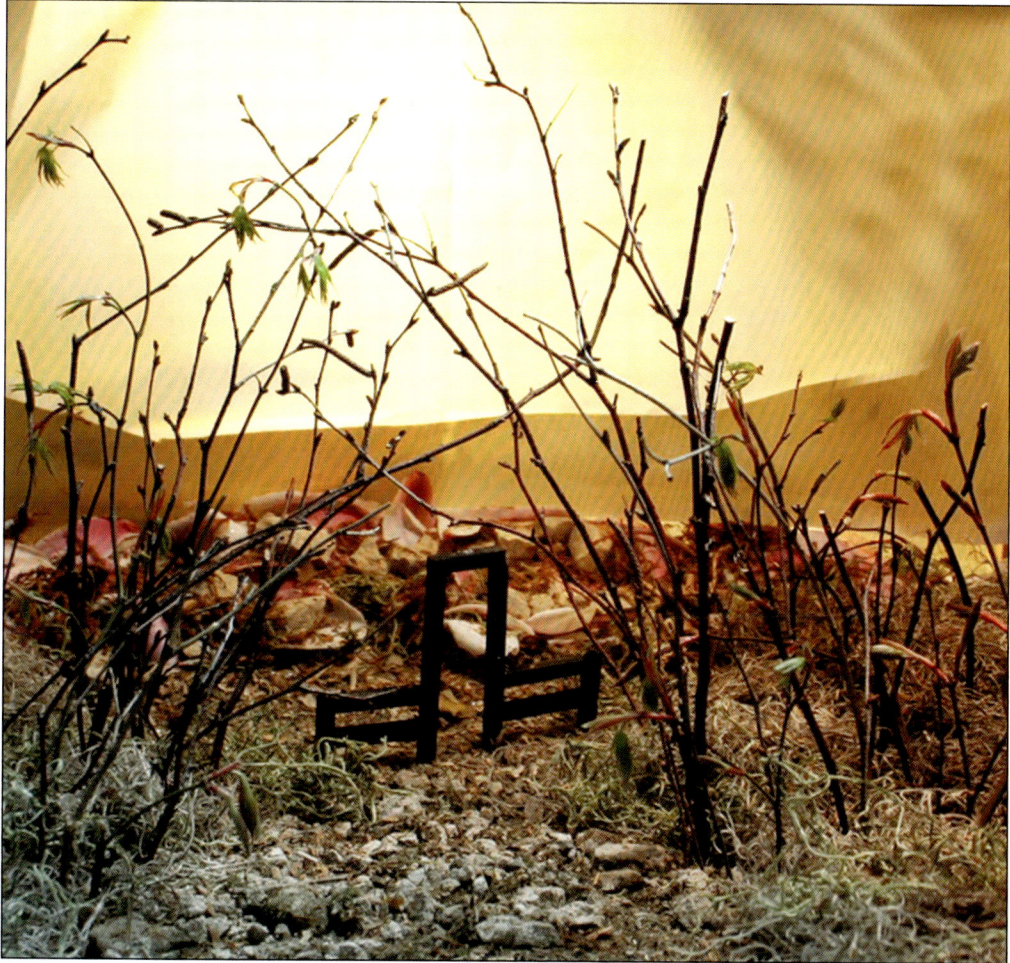

Gate Memoryscape, diorama

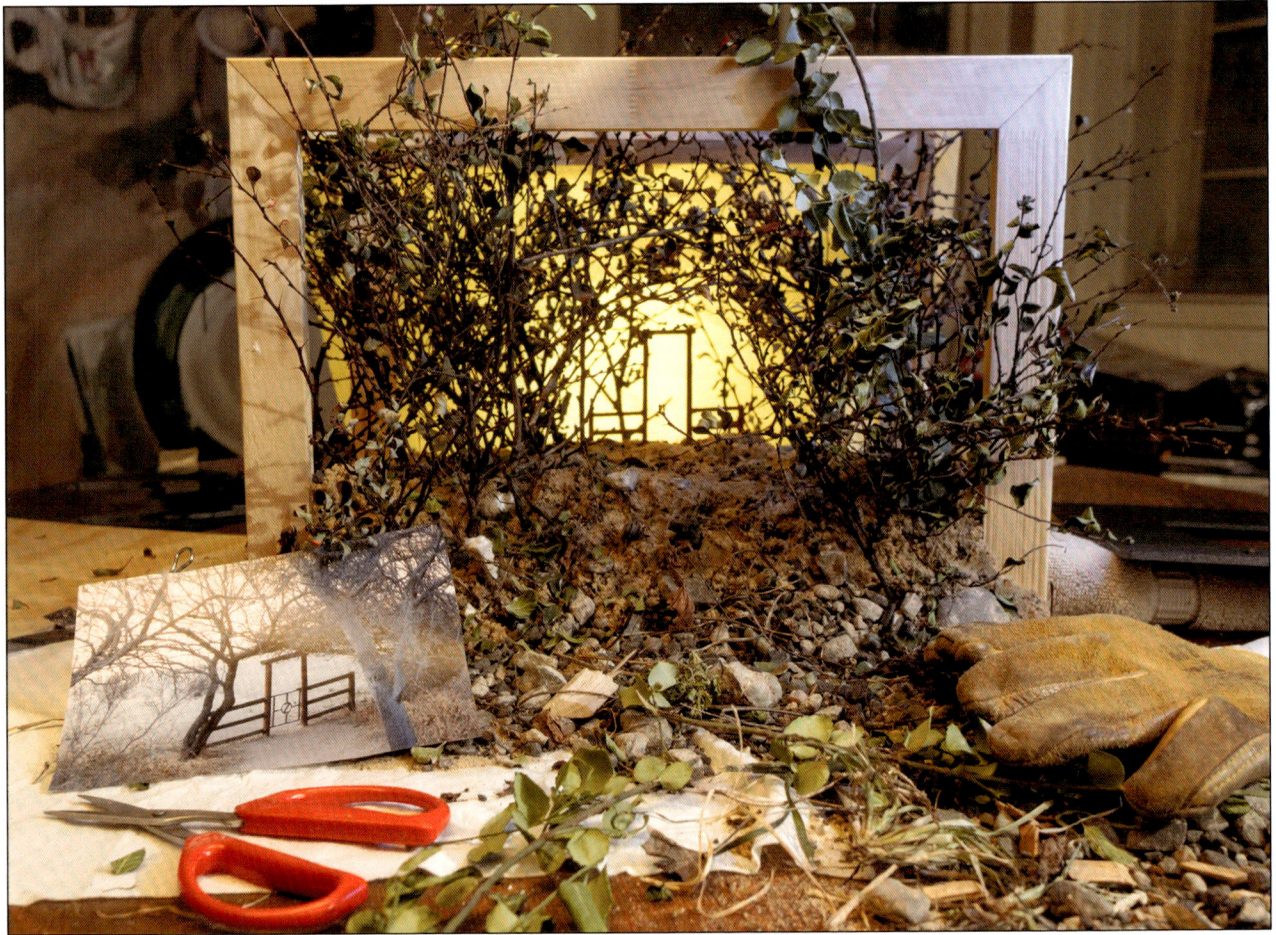

Gate Memoryscape, diorama

markable places on the ranch. I took photographs at different times of day, in different light, from different angles, tight and wide. These adjustments produced detailed photographs that looked like focused replicas of the sites but nevertheless were poor likenesses of the "real" mental images Clearly, these memoryscapes were always destined to remain neither here nor there. I wanted to understand what of the here shaped the there and why the memoryscapes were so accessible to my mind's eye as freshly particular yet partially abstracted images. I began to immerse myself more deeply in the landscapes of the memoryscapes by spending more time each day at the actual sites without a camera, just looking. They responded to me, saying, "Yes, yes, you're right, I do come from here. This is my earthly birthplace, but I can never entirely be from here." So I began to make drawings to see if those captured the look of the memoryscapes more accurately. I attempted to draw the memoryscapes as I looked at the actual landscape from which they came. During those afternoons I also wrote down a detailed description of what I saw. These accounts, while good for describing details of the view, seemed to slice the memoryscapes into little unrelated pieces, making them even more difficult to capture. I felt as if the words were tearing the image apart and turning it into thin strips of paper. I returned to Philadelphia with a lot to look at and think about. I knew how to call up the memoryscapes, look at them, hold them steady in view, and visually enter their deeper space. I found refuge in them and moved outward from their interior spaces to have new experiences each time I viewed them, but I could not adequately describe them.

In Philadelphia, I set up a workspace and began experimenting with the photographs and drawings to see if I could build the memoryscapes in three dimensions. Unlike the dioramas, they were two-dimensional flat views and only became three-dimensional within a very limited interior space once I visually entered them. In building a three-dimensional replica, I transformed the memoryscapes into dioramas. With the crude effects of balsa wood, paint, colored gels, bits of earth, and paper cutouts, I built miniature dioramas and photographed them. These homemade constructions came the closest to capturing what I saw before me when I looked deeply into the memoryscapes. The multiple views of the Gate Diorama in the photograph I took show the transformation of space that I perceived once my imagination was activated. The Corral Diorama photographs emphasize how the sky appeared to descend directly down onto the ground, pressing down onto the horses as if there were no earthly natural environment between them and the sky.

One time, however, reality coincided with the magical presence I felt in seeing memoryscapes materialize in the photographs I took of the mini-dioramas. This occurred on November 2, 2017. To the northeast, where the horizon met the Patagonia Mountains, an enlarged, fast-rising, nearly-full moon emerged right at their base and barreled down toward me. This immense orb filled the sky directly overhead on its accelerating rise. It was a Beaver Moon, also known as a Hunters Moon, just shy of the super moon that would appear a few days later when the full moon would be closer to the earth than at any other time of the year. This giant loomed over the earth, elbowing aside twilight and the tranquility it brings before nightfall. Standing helpless under it, I felt precariously perched at the midpoint of a tilting seesaw that flung the huge moon into the sky. It was as if the landscape itself became a memoryscape, making the heavens swirl. The earth felt as if it hiccupped around me as the moon pressed down upon it. It was like a magical visual intrusion similar to the effect of a memoryscape. The distorted moon reminded me that the native geography from which a memoryscape originated can be disrupted.

I returned again to the ranch in 2006, 2008, 2010, 2013, and 2017. As I continued to explore how the memoryscapes came to be and why they worked, I began to realize how much they reminded me of dioramas. They were cousins of sorts. The memoryscape's deep space reminded me of the multiple planes of view in the unrolling landscapes painted on the background walls of the dioramas. The taxidermied animals stood in the foreground, life-sized and looking out into vast expanses, just as I did when entering a memoryscapes, and like them I found myself caught in a timeless moment in a three-dimensional space where I was free to view the scene and also have my own simultaneous experience. And most remarkable, when I entered the deep space of a diorama or a memoryscape, I no longer felt like that person split in two by migraine disease. The more I became a part of the surrounding landscape, the more I felt whole.[1]

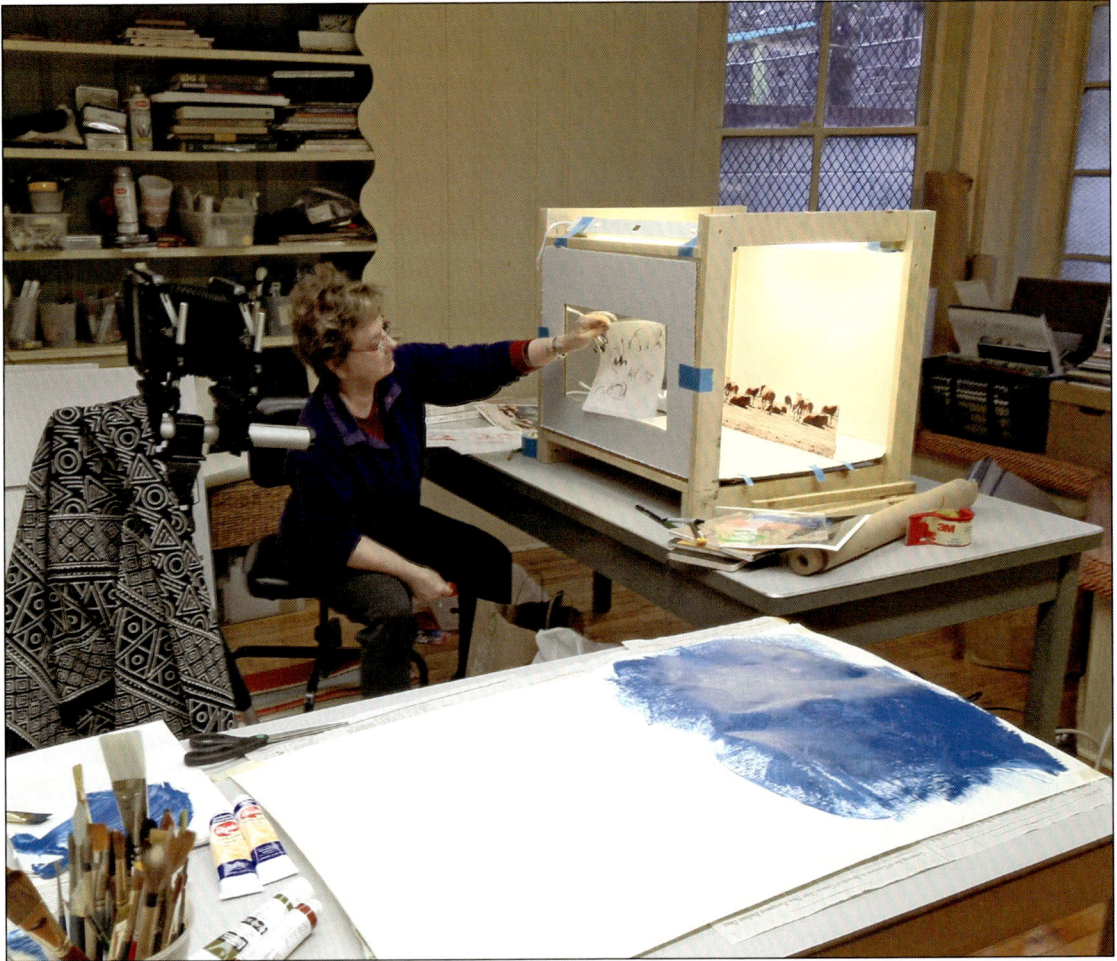

Building a Diorama

CHAPTER FIVE

NEAR GUAYMAS

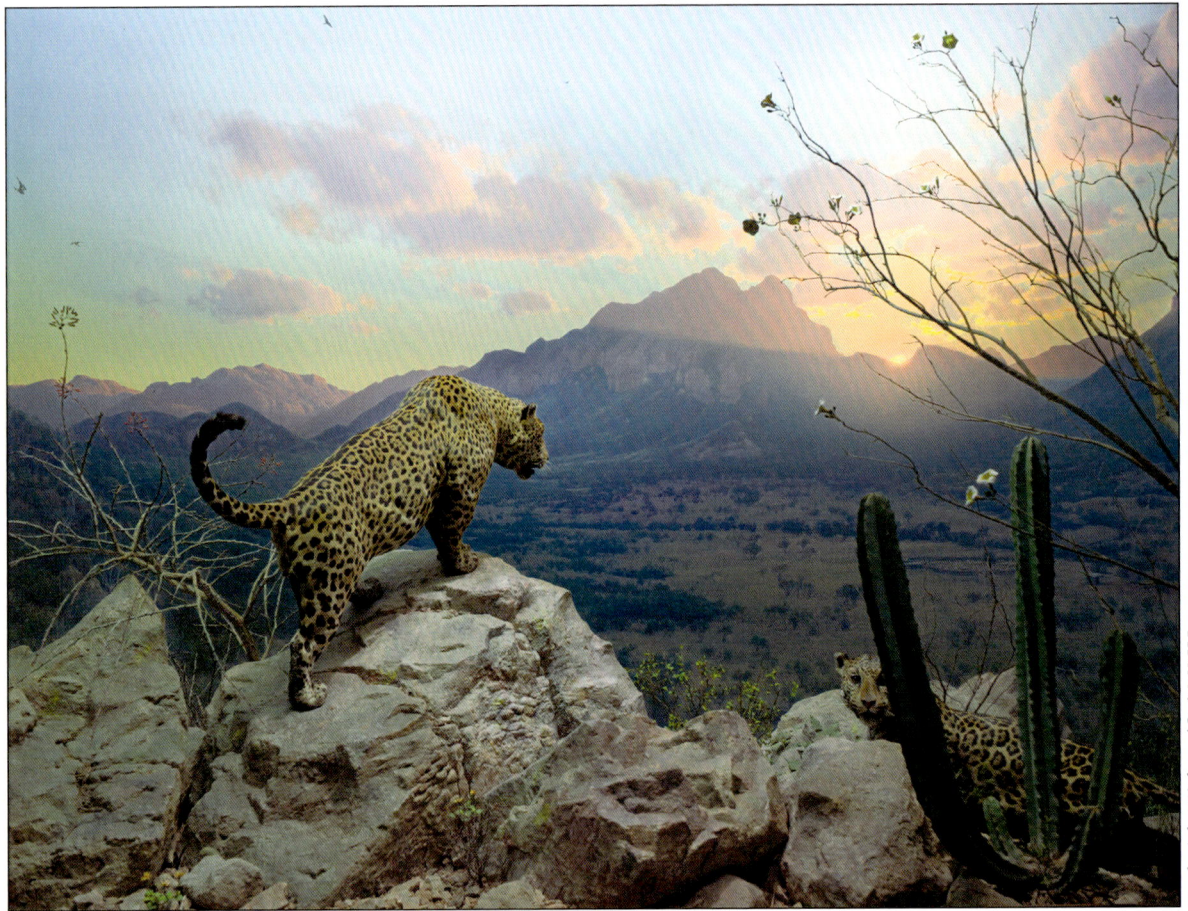

Jaguar Diorama, The Bernard Family Hall of North American Mammals,
American Museum of Natural History

J ust as the big jaguar steps up onto a rocky outcrop, the October sun begins to set. The colors suffusing the sky and clouds above are as striking as the patterns on his coat. The last slanting rays of light from the setting sun sink behind the distant mountains and transform the Sonoran Desert into shades of rose and dark green. Twilight descends on the valley below as the jaguar looks down into it. In this diorama the plate glass window seems inadequate as a barrier between us and this apex predator. He leans forward on padded front paws that bear the weight of his lowered head and muscular shoulders. His graceful up-curved tail steadies his hind legs while he tenses both ears, drops open his jaw, and looks further into the graying landscape. Dusk fades quickly here in the desert. In the distance, livestock begin to rustle within a makeshift corral. It is unclear whether they are settling down for the night or moving about because they sense imminent danger. Just now, the jaguar has emerged from the daytime cover of the enclosed canyon behind him. The air is cooler now and his night vision is sharper.

Partially hidden among the rocks at his side, his mate, or perhaps his sibling, is at rest, but alert. She faces us. When her mild, wide-eyed gaze meets ours, she seems more surprised than threatened. We and she are bound together, each arrested in this moment of direct contact. Her soft ears frame an intricate design of spots arrayed across her forehead. Larger rosettes form cube-shaped patterns with black insets and brown centers that cascade down her back and reach the tip of her tail. Her coat blends seamlessly with the rocks and desert plants surrounding her. Although the drama of the hunt is embodied by the male, her awareness of us heightens the tension of the diorama. Her strong gaze holds us captive. As long as we remain immobile, she allows us access to this scene by not turning to alert her mate to our presence. He, she, and we array ourselves at the base of a triangle whose hypotenuse opens onto the drama this diorama suggests. From our position, we take in the whole diorama. We see the two jaguars slightly ahead of us, and then we look outward into the middle and far distance, to the mountains at this dramatic sunset. It creates this brief moment of nightly synchrony emerging between animal and element. At first the fearsome jaguar with his downward gaze rivets us, then we become aware that his head is in direct alignment with the setting sun, the other equally powerful subject of this diorama.

To the west, wispy, fracto-cumulous clouds, illuminated in graduated shades of pale yellow, pink, and violet, dip toward the mountains and appear to be sucked down into the funnel of bright orange light that transects the mountains where the sun is setting. The changing colors of the atmosphere flood the desert landscape. High above, the clear sky ranges in color from pale yellow and white at the horizon upward into violet and then changes to a deep cobalt blue at the apex. Lower, where the sun is setting, a shaft of intense light illuminates the distant mountains. The top third of the mountains glows red, the bottom two thirds deepen to shades of violet, then lower down the slopes become blue, and finally the muted greens and browns of the valley floor. The pale gray tones of twilight begin to drain color from the trees and scrubland in the near distance. Right now, the remaining sliver of the sun is about to disappear, and when it does, the jaguar's coat will suddenly fade, for it, as well, is flecked with reflected light. The whole valley will darken. Our imaginary foothold on the rocks will become less secure. All implied action will alter as this one charged moment vanishes.

I visually enter the diorama from my position high up in the canyon rocks. There I scan the terrain, looking for a place to travel deeper into it. Down below in the valley, the fading light softens the edges of the scrub and makes the patches of oak and mesquite appear bluer while dulling the yellow color of the valley's grasses. I follow the sightlines of the jaguar. I make out a continuous line of trees snaking across the land: perhaps they are cottonwoods that border a constantly flowing stream that provides water year-round to this part of the valley. The Sonoita creek at the ranch comes to mind. I begin to descend into the valley. My ankles itch from the scratching of rough grasses, even though I know they still are pliable and not as parched as they will become after the new year. Now I can see the outlines of the circular makeshift corral and attached sheds, which the jaguar spots with ease. This corral is an actual representation of the refuge I seek deep in the middle distance of each of my memoryscapes. But here in the Jaguar Diorama, the livestock enclosure suggests the opposite of safety: it concentrates the jaguar's prey in a vulnerable place. Nevertheless, I am strongly drawn to this ramshackle corral. To my troubled brain this space, placed within the surrounding landscape of the diorama, promises refuge. It is the only corral I see in all the dioramas I visit in the museum and it is set in the very same landscape as Circle Z. I am at ease now, though I know full well the diorama means to tell a different tale.

I first view the jaguars close up, in a flat, two-dimensional plane. This frontal view allows me to measure myself in relation to them, an experience I would never have with an apex predator in real life. Beyond them, the landscape unrolls in three-dimensional linear perspective. Our ability to simultaneously experience both flat frontal and then three-dimensional perspectival space allows us to first step into the diorama and visually inhabit it before we begin to move forward, deeper into the interior. The foreground where the jaguar stands joins the painted background just below the steep drop-off that lies beyond the rocks. The valley below is framed east to west by the distant mountains and by the foreground rocks. This framing slightly compresses the view in the middle distance. Here, multiple focal planes formed by horizontal lines of desert scrub and trees guide me into and across the landscape. In the valley I begin to lose the long view that contains both jaguar and sunset. From a different perspective the drama of the hunt vanishes. The space I am in now becomes the container for another set of observations and imaginary experiences.

The jaguar finds himself frozen in a fast-changing moment, as fast as the familiar setting sun that descends beyond him. He and the rose-tinted sunset compete equally for my attention. The jaguar, a beautiful, massive mounted specimen, embodies the best natural science offers museum displays; the sunset is a marvel of landscape painting. With an exactitude originating in precise observation and superior artistic rendering of the site, the background painting sets the mood and heightens the illusion of reality. James Perry Wilson (1889–1976), the background painter, was a master at painting landscapes on the difficult domed, curved background walls of dioramas. Between 1938 and 1954 he painted nineteen of the twenty-nine dioramas in the Hall of North American Mammals, as well as six in the Akeley Hall of African Mammals. Like other background painters, he used a combination of painted panoramic references, photographs, and scaled models, as well as direct field observation. What made him so outstanding was his ability to paint light's effect on the atmosphere and the landscape. His mastery of linear and aerial perspective anchors objects in space and makes vast distances credible. Wilson's backgrounds presented more accurately what the eye sees on the ground than what the world looks like viewed as a painting or photograph. The dimensionality of the background painting in the Jaguar

Diorama guarantees that I feel I am there, securely within the landscape when I pass through the glass. The innovative grids Wilson invented and projected on the back wall as guides to his painting were unequal in size, being slightly curved at the edges to extend the even plane of the viewing area in a manner that compensated for the distortion caused by the curve of the walls. In the Jaguar Diorama, the distant mountains extend outward across the horizon and wrap only slightly toward us at the sides to meet our gaze.

When Wilson arrived at the museum in 1934 he was already a skilled architectural draftsman and designer, as well as an accomplished plein air painter. Soon he would become famous for the breathtaking light infused blue skies he created by blending bands of color in premixed tints to create the seamless progressions that descended from the highest point in the sky down to the horizon line. That accomplished, he moved forward and painted from the horizon toward the foreground. Unlike other background painters, he did not manipulate the landscape to create harmonious compositions; his goal was fidelity to what he saw at the site.

To achieve the luminous sky in the Jaguar Diorama he used a technique called scumbling, in which he combined gentle horizontal and vertical brush strokes to make the edges disappear between the sections of color he wished to join together. In the sky, we see violet and rose-tinted light reflected onto the denser undersides of the wispy clouds rushing westward toward the sunset. As we look down toward the sunset from the highest point in the sky, blue light is filtered out and replaced at the lower altitudes by a wash of the rich reddish tones that spread over the mountains. Hidden from public view, five incandescent spotlights direct additional light at the sun while keeping the valley and foreground darker. The fast-moving clouds and the low angle of the sun's rays create the sense of motion and drama in this arrested moment. The jaguar is caught one way in this moment and we viewers another; for us, our sense of wonder at this brief radiance co-exists with our awareness of its predatory significance for the jaguar. What he makes of this splendor we know not.

Wilson began working on the Jaguar Diorama in 1942. However, he did not actually visit the site of this box canyon near Guaymas in Western Sonora, Mexico. Instead, he used Bernard Chapman's studies as his working references. Chapman had already begun the diorama when he left the museum at the approach of the war, as many did. Wilson took over. He rethought the diorama's presentation and chose to strengthen its impact by changing the original early morning setting to a dramatic sunset. He based this change on a black and white photograph of the site whose angle of view is duplicated in the finished painting. To design the background he used both Chapman's painted and photographic references, although he ultimately preferred the photographic references. His goal, however, was never to produce a purely photographic rendering of the site. He achieved depth and mood through drawing and painting. First, Wilson drew the entire background in charcoal before applying paint. His backgrounds are much better aligned with what the human eye actually sees. Sunsets became a signature of Wilson's work. He finished the Jaguar Diorama in early 1943 and hurried on to the Mule Deer.

There are no empty spaces in a good diorama, no such thing as no place at all. No cosmic emptiness fills its habitat. Dioramas such as the ones in New York always record a real place. Everything within the Jaguar Diorama is interconnected to create a seamless landscape, just as all the parts of a good painting make sense, edge to edge, up close and far away. If the diorama is not well executed in all its constructed and painted parts, the illusion of reality fails and the life of the moment it depicts is not credible.

At first glance, the livestock enclosure in the Jaguar Diorama is easy to miss; it sits in the distance off to the right and appears vague in the hazy twilight, bracketed by two arms of an imposing cactus in the foreground. It comes into sharper focus as I move closer to it. Only by following the jaguar's gaze does the viewer seek it out. As I begin to approach it now from my position down in the low grasses, its oblong shape becomes clearer. On the side facing me, a wide gate is shut now that the livestock have entered for the night. The fence is made of irregularly placed mesquite stakes, roughly bound together with heavy baling wire. To my left, the corral opens at one end into a low circular shed with a covered roof where the feed is probably kept. In the middle of the corral the livestock gather around a solitary tree. Outside the corral and a little way off to the right, another shed with an exterior overhanging roof looks as if it were used either for extra storage or for human shelter. In the quiet and muted twilight I see no sign of anyone attending to the livestock. The land on which the corral sits is in no way disturbed by the imposition of these few structures upon it.

For me, refuge from pain means, above all, a safe place. The undulating fence encloses just the right size space I seek. Within the corral's confines, shelter allows re-orientation. Each refuge within a memoryscape or a diorama requires some edge that delineates the safe space within. These refuges are found deep within the middle distances of the landscape. The irregular, oblong shape of this corral and its loose, roughly-made mesquite fence offer just enough containment. Its curving outline follows the natural contours of a terrain similar to the ranch's. I recognize the land around me as being the same shape as the Patagonia mountains. In here, I recall how I used to come upon old corrals such as these, either abandoned or still used. Looking up into the sky, the distant jaguar and the sunset appear very far away, almost non-existent. It's as if they are perched on opposite outer edges of a large circular container comprising the dome of the diorama. Soon I feel like I do when I enter those deep places of refuge in the memoryscapes. The menacing void of a migraine is replaced by the rich particulars of the world around me. Soon I am creating my own stories of life in this valley.

In the early 1940s, Bernard Chapman and his museum colleagues visited a box canyon located about two hundred and eighty miles southwest of Circle Z, to the east of Guaymas,

Sonora, in the Sonoran Desert in northern Mexico. There they made studies, took photographs, and collected plant specimens for the Jaguar Diorama. They also captured and shipped the jaguar to New York. Although jaguars once ranged as far north as the Grand Canyon, in the mid twentieth century, jaguar sightings were infrequent. By then jaguars had been hunted almost to extinction. Not until 1996 were they listed as an endangered species. Jaguars range widely; they move northward over the wooded slopes of the Sky Island ranges that surround Circle Z, through grasslands, deserts, and mountains in search of new breeding grounds. Currently a stable population of about two hundred cats resides about a hundred miles south of the border. Males from this group are increasingly being seen in southern Arizona. In 2009, a male jaguar named Macho B was sighted south of Tucson on the eastern slopes of the Santa Ritas, northwest of Circle Z. In 2015, El Jefe was photographed, also in the Santa Ritas after having been previously spotted in 2011, less than thirty miles south of Tucson, within range of the proposed Rosemont open pit copper mine. Remarkably, he was photographed again in November of 2021 in central Sonora, having successfully negotiated the border wall. In 2016 and 2017 a cat named Yo'oko Nahsuareo was photographed by camera traps in the Huachucas, about twenty-five miles to the east of the ranch. Currently one male jaguar resides in the Chiricahua mountains close to the border.

Jaguars have been impeded in their movements into Arizona both by the two hundred and ten miles of the border wall constructed in Arizona during the Trump administration and by road construction accompanying the building and maintenance of the entire wall. Habitat destruction, proposed massive mining sites, population growth, degradation of water resources, and prey depletion further lessen their chances of successfully establishing new breeding grounds. However, in 2020 a juvenile male, Bonito, was spotted less than sixty miles from the border in Sonora, on a ranch owned by a Sonoran-based conservation organization. His presence there is a good indication that breeding populations of jaguars are beginning to move north. The mountains where jaguars have been seen—the Patagonias, the Santa Ritas, and the Huachucas—are islands of viable habitat, connected by the same deserts and grasslands that encircle the ranch.

The Jaguar Diorama, finished in 1943, depicts the uneasy relationship between this apex predator and the cattle ranchers working in the Sonoran grasslands. This relationship is changing today. A program called Viviendo con Felinos (Living with Felines), which is part of the Northern Jaguar Project, pays ranchers in Sonora much like those in the area of Guaymas to photograph jaguars with camera traps instead of hunting them, making it far more lucrative to collect a fee for each camera trap photo. Urgent conservation efforts are increasing on both sides of the border, although jaguars continue to encounter many threats to their survival: availability of prey, poaching, proposed mining developments, and habitat destruction all limit the possibility of their expansion northward.

With the re-appearance of jaguars in the Sky Island ranges, the jaguar in the Jaguar Diorama suddenly shed a new light on the ranch. After a lifetime, the ranch has been jostled from its position in my mind as the reassuring, unchanging landscape of childhood memory. One day, as I stood looking at the jaguar in the museum, he seemed to burst forth out of the timeless, static container of his glass-enclosed diorama and appear massive and alive, beside a living contemporary counterpart, struggling in the fluid, changing present. They stood together as siblings in the Sonoran habitat they once could depend on. At that moment I began to understand the ranch differently. I became aware of how frozen it had become in my mind, of how I had taken its geography for granted as an unchanging landscape of my memory. Because of the jaguar sightings, the Patagonias could no longer be viewed as an undisturbed habitat in an unchanging geographical setting, and this knowledge shook the foundation on which my abstracted memoryscapes rested. I saw before me the present, roiling with the potential impact of the proposed Hermosa-South 32 mine, only six miles south of Patagonia: an open pit, 4,000-foot wide, 1,500-foot deep, silver, lead, manganese, and zinc mine that would move over a thousand times more rock than the largest of any of the past Patagonia mines. If dug, it would be one of the largest zinc mines in the world. Road building, ground water pumping, water contamination and the transportation of ore would alter the landscape for the fifty-year duration of the proposed mineral extraction. The ecological impact of this would irrevocably change this hunting ground for the jaguar, alter the quality of life in Patagonia, affect the land and water in the surrounding areas, and could call into question the ranch's future. Already on the ranch's own 6,500 acres, many plant and animal species were becoming vulnerable to climate change.

The Jaguar Diorama, Circle Z Ranch, and the memoryscapes all converged. My understanding of place changed, and the grip my memory and imagination had on the memoryscapes loosened.[1]

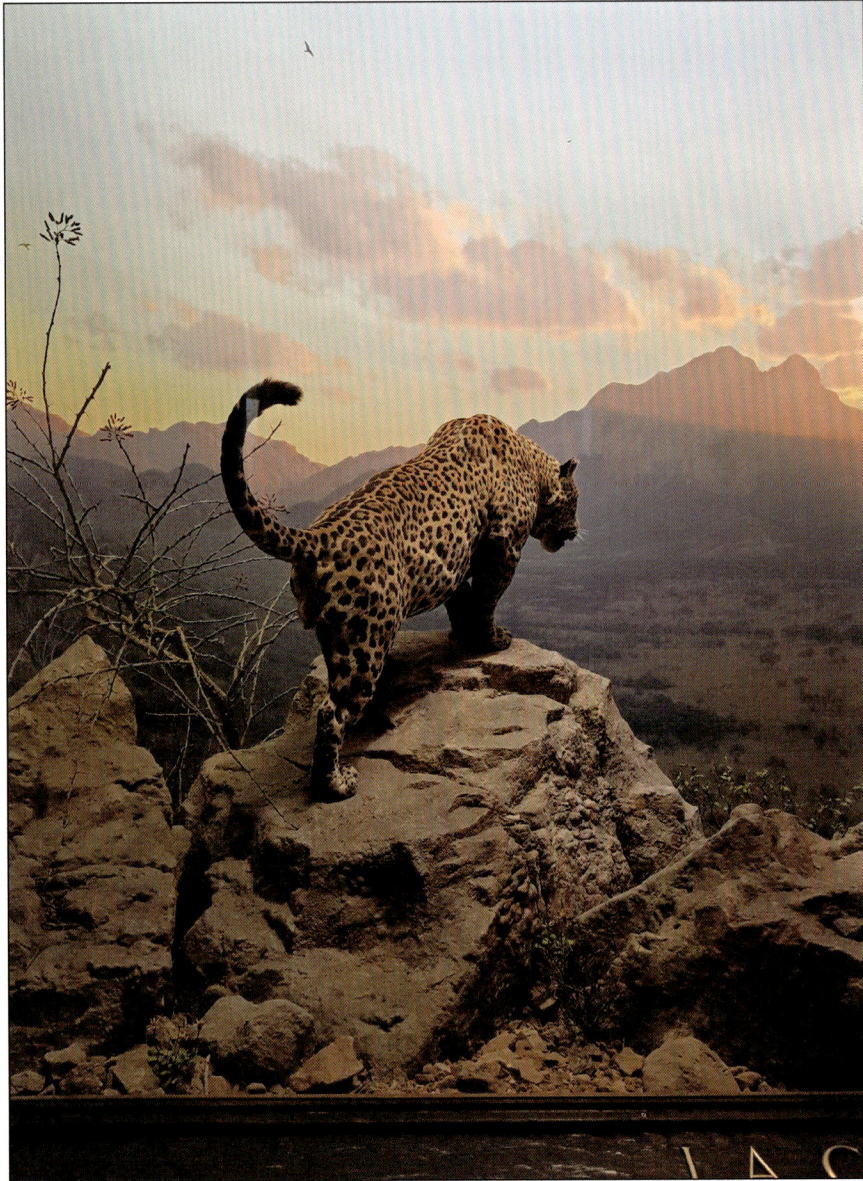

Jaguar at Risk

CHAPTER SIX

AT YOSEMITE

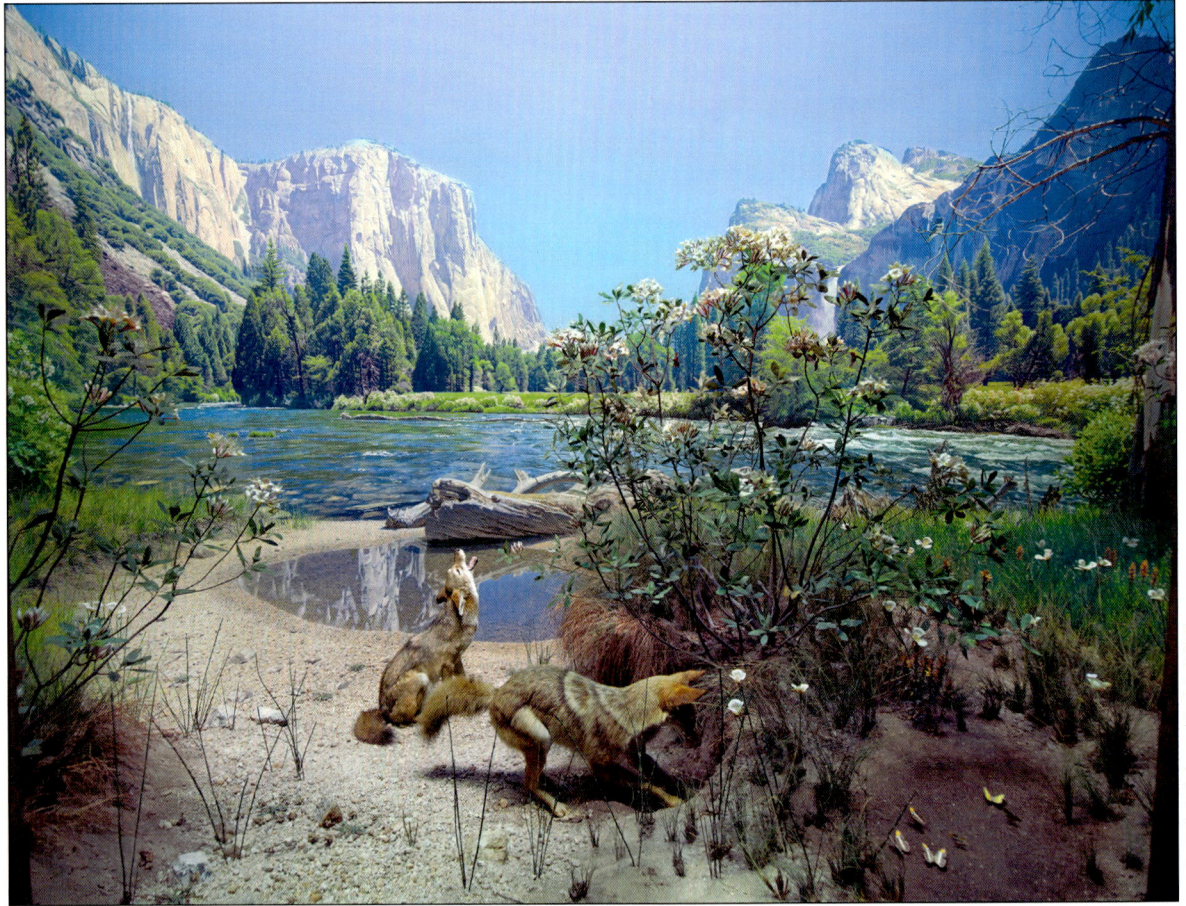

Coyote Diorama, The Bernard Family Hall of North American Mammals,
American Museum of Natural History

U pon entering the Akeley Hall, the viewer steps into one of the darkest areas in the museum. This is the roughly twenty-foot-wide space between the extraordinary group of eight mounted African elephants titled "The Alarm" in the Hall's center and the dioramas that surround them. After the glare of the Roosevelt Rotunda, this disorienting darkness is not accidental. Once inside, one feels as if a heavy black curtain has fallen for an instant, much like a circus flap, and then has been pulled back to reveal a dazzling glimpse of twenty-eight glowing dioramas. A dramatic scene within the big tent of science, education, and entertainment opens before the viewer. As its own place, the Hall is spectacular. Everything about its art deco design focuses the viewer's attention on the jewel-like eighteen-foot-high dioramas that line the walls on the ground and mezzanine levels. These forty-foot-high walls are covered in dark green serpentine. Creating a border at the top of the dioramas, beautiful bronze relief friezes link the African scenes below. Each display is named with a bronze label at its base. Wall text is kept to a minimum and placed discreetly to one side.

Carl Akeley, a master taxidermist, hunter, sculptor, and innovator, was the visionary creator of this magnificent exhibit space. He conceived of the hall in 1909, but it did not open until 1936, ten years after his death, and it was not fully completed until 1942. Akeley demanded that each item made for the dioramas, whether a mounted specimen or a replica of a plant or geologic feature, be scientifically accurate. He also understood the importance of the background paintings as indispensable artistic components for communicating the scenic magnificence of Africa and as well as depicting the habitats of the mammals.

The twenty-eight habitat dioramas in the Hall are natural history scenarios. They contain three-dimensional full-scale mounted specimens of mammals placed in their native surroundings, behind which painted landscapes on curved alcoves extend the foreground scene into the surrounding African landscape. These dioramas are not just for viewing the accurate scenes they portray. At the same time that the viewer looks at their convincing realistic detail, he may also imaginatively enter their interior space. This simultaneous viewing of the diorama "reality" along with imaginative parallel immersion is often what adults remember most about their first experiences at the museum. Being there resides in their memories alongside memories of the size of the immense cloak room.

Dioramas are pristine environments, devoid of humans and ever available as spaces for sustained viewing. Inside, the plants, trees, rocks, and fallen leaves are eternally fresh, just as the stopped moment in which we find ourselves is always avail-

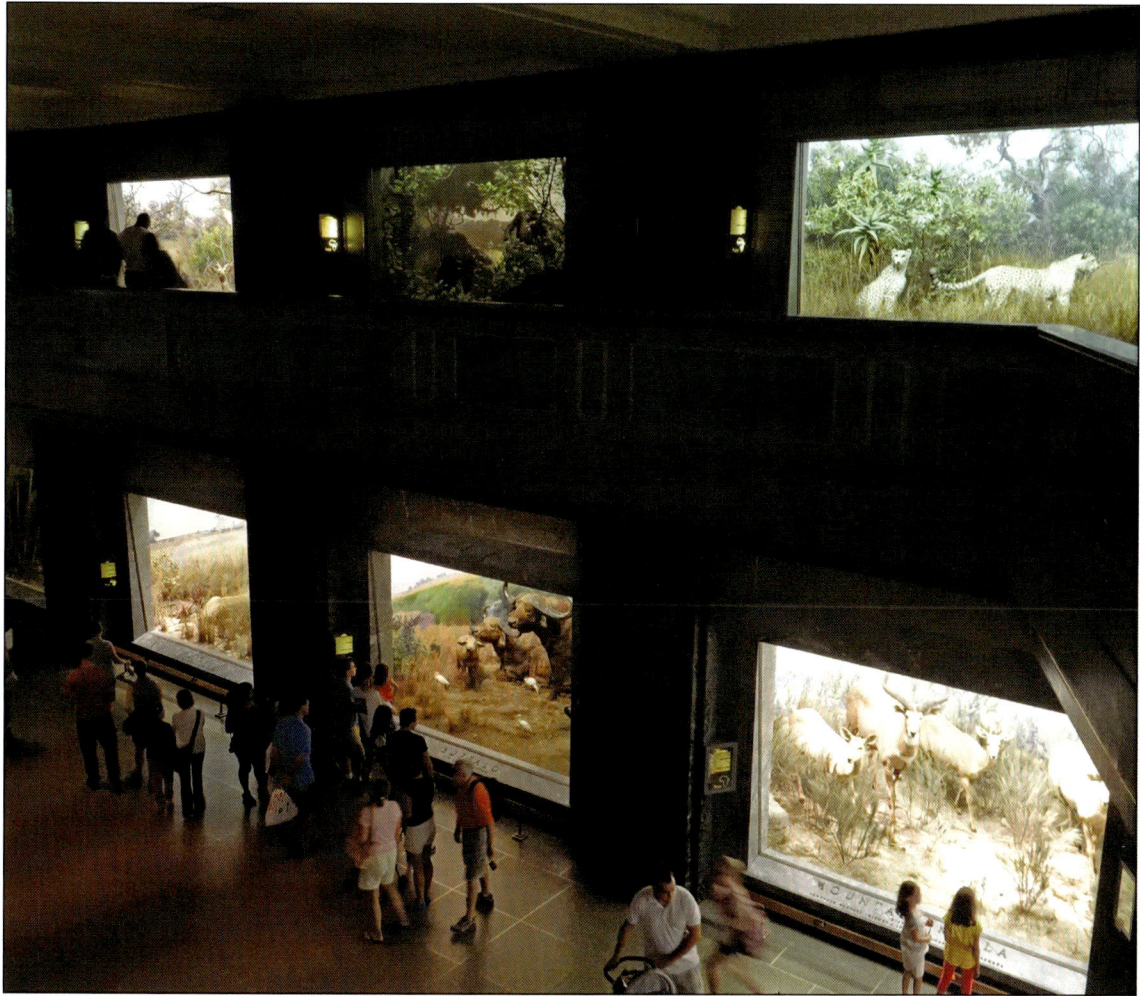

Akeley Hall of African Mammals, American Museum of Natural History

able for potential discovery. The Akeley Hall is the first place I visit when I come to the museum. Sights unimaginable and unseen by the American viewer at the time of its the construction still retain their power to enthrall me, even though I know them well through other mediums and their groupings in some instances have been subject to scientific revision.

The Akeley Hall of African Mammals and the Hall of North American Mammals house twenty-eight dioramas and fifty-seven dioramas, respectively. Each diorama is set behind a slanted, clear, plate glass viewing window and is illuminated from within by concealed lights. Their painted, curved walls connect to the three-dimensional foreground. Mounted specimens of mammals are surrounded by artificial vegetation, earth and rocks. All dioramas ideally are viewed without the mediation of technical devices such as still cameras or moving picture cameras, which alter the size and shape of what they portray as well as the viewing planes. Some dioramas are set below ground level in order to create a slight drop in elevation that further enhances the illusion of infinite space receding into the distance, a feature strikingly different from memoryscapes in which the perception of infinite space rises directly upward, often from the middle distance. Other dioramas are placed slightly above ground to create the impression of a steep drop to the space into which the viewer looks.

At its founding in 1869, the American Museum of Natural History dedicated itself to "advancing the general knowledge of kindred subjects and to the end of furnishing popular instruction and education."[1] Unlike its European counterparts, the museum's purpose added this function to collection and research. This shift to a belief that the education of people in a democratic society is an important mission for a natural history museum was foreshadowed at the founding, eighty-three years earlier in 1786, of the first popular private American museum of natural science, Peale's Philadelphia Museum. It contained many early examples of what, in the late nineteenth century and early twentieth century, developed into modern diorama displays. These displays resembled miniature cabinets of curiosities in that they were cases, stacked one atop another along the walls of a long gallery.

Today, Charles Willson Peale's grand 1822 self portrait, "The Artist in the Museum," vividly illustrates the design and purpose of a natural history museum. His imposing form fills the foreground; his right arm pulls back a heavy, fringed, russet-colored velvet curtain that covers most of the upper half of the eight-foot-high painting. Behind this curtain, a long gallery containing rows of diorama cases filled with stuffed birds displayed against primitive painted backdrops extends back to the rear wall, above which hang portraits of dignitaries and scientists. Four patrons of the museum stand in front of the cases and admire the display. The closest to the viewer, a woman in the middle distance, raises her arms in a gesture of delight as she gazes across the gallery; farther on, a man stands next to his son, who is taking notes as he studies the birds; and in the background another man is absorbed in contemplation. Peale's audience is the same one sought by the designers of the Akeley Hall. In front of Peale, in the lower left foreground, a stuffed wild turkey extends its long neck and beak downward to inspect a box that contains an array of Peale's taxidermy tools. In the right foreground, a mastodon jaw provides a spectacular draw for visitors. Next to it, two long bones rest on the edge of a table draped in heavy green cloth on which also sits Peale's palette and brushes. These two balanced elements make clear the crucial collaboration between taxidermy, natural science, and art that are still crucial to the success of modern dioramas. The museum's mission is to "bring into view a world in miniature"[2] and to do it in a way that would "please and entertain the public."[3] Carl Akeley, 105 years later, extended Peale's vision. Unlike the enduring African Hall, the collection of 10,000 specimens in Peale's Museum was dispersed and finally sold in 1849 to Phineas T. Barnum and Moses Kimball. It went the way of the public's desire for entertainment over education, favoring circus spectacles and side show oddities. The gigantic mastodon bones seen behind Peale drew the crowds into the gallery, just as the elephants do in the Akeley Hall.

Today, dioramas no longer serve the crowds in quite the same way as in their heyday in the early twentieth century. By the 1950s, animal documentaries and other film technologies brought the public in close contact with the animals and the places portrayed in most dioramas. But it was not so a century ago for Carl Akeley. These products of ambitious hunting and collecting expeditions to faraway places thrilled New Yorkers.

Although the habitat dioramas constructed by Akeley in the early twentieth century differ significantly in form and content from Louis Daguerre's nineteenth-century precursors, they bear the stamp of Daguerre's creations from which they get their name. In both, the viewer looks into a life-sized, three-dimensional construction to see a scene that is made dramatic and realistic by the use of artificial lighting, painted backdrops, and masterfully-placed objects. In Daguerre's dioramas, however, lighting and other effects moved, altering what the viewer saw while he viewed them. Both Daguerre's and the AMNH's constructions conform in spirit to the Latin meaning of the word "diorama," which is derived from two roots: *dia*, meaning "through," and *horao*, meaning "view."

Dioramas and memoryscapes are both similar and different, just as cousins may bear a family resemblance but look quite different. Memoryscapes fill my field of view, just as dioramas do. Dioramas, however, unlike memoryscapes, are both two- and three-dimensional. Their foregrounds, though actually three-dimensional, can be read as flat and two-dimensional when we view them up close on one plane, while the backgrounds—which are actually two-dimensional—are understood as three-dimensional. Memoryscapes look two-dimensional all over until we enter their limited protected spaces and our imagination takes over. Memoryscapes have a hyper-real, vaguely pointillistic quality, yet dioramas are so real and natural looking to the eye that the viewer willingly suspends her disbelief. Memoryscapes, although derived from reality, are never entirely real looking. They are imagination-made. Habitat dioramas never are.

How is it possible that the vast landscape of Yosemite, with such a vibrant sense of motion and depth, can be so credibly contained beyond a plate glass window within a box? The Coyote Diorama in the Hall of North American Mammals bursts into our field of view, radiating an explosive energy from all surfaces. At Valley View we encounter a perfect summer day in the Yosemite Valley. The sky is a deep blue above the Merced River, which rushes by in the near distance and moves so rapidly that white caps break its surface. Reflections of brilliant mid-morning light glance off the sparkling water. In the foreground a coyote points its open, white muzzle skyward to yip and yap in what looks to be full-throated exuberance that broadcasts the presence of his pack. To his right, his companion extends its tail and aims its ears forward while vigorously pawing the moist gravel in hopes of perhaps unearthing a gopher. Far off, the massive El Capitan looms, rising near the horizon. Close to the viewing window, a large rhododendron bush with mariposa lilies fills the right half of the diorama with white flowering buds that open toward the sunlight. This tall plant is the entry point into the diorama as well as a counterbalance to its vast vista. The distance from the coyotes to the mountain is immense. So far is the enormous granite face of the mountain, it looks pale in comparison with the other closer yet still distant mountains and trees. The two coyotes cavort on a gravel sand bar beside a shallow reflecting pool in the foreground, an addition on James Perry Wilson's part, in which El Capitan's reflection is also visible. Beyond them, a hollowed out bleached log sits at the river's edge. A meadow borders the opposite bank, and farther still a semicircle of enormous fir trees creates a wall that bisects the scene and anchors El Capitan. Across a broad valley, closer to the viewer, more mountains rise. The Bridal Veil Falls cascade down the slopes on the right. Unlike the Jaguar Diorama in which we and the jaguar both look into the valley below, here the scene is so vast it is left to us to try to comprehend it. The coyotes don't look directly into it to guide us. Instead, they exist as their own unit within its vastness, integral to its wild beauty but only directly occupied with a small portion of the scene. The menace and drama of an apex predator is replaced here by the coyotes' vigorous activity, the energy of the river, and the vastness and vitality of the landscape.

As visually active as this diorama is, I still find within it a number of calming sources of visual refuge; the shallow pool, the meadow, the protecting curve of the fir trees, and even the bordered confines of the fast-moving river provide a protected space for me to visually enter as I move deeper into Yosemite. The active world swirls around these protected spaces, and its forceful presence and immense three-dimensional scale beckon the viewer inside. I find refuge from pain in a number of these spaces deep within this scene.

The Circle Z Mountain Memoryscape is as quiet as the Coyote Diorama is active. The mountain that occupies most of this memoryscape dominates the view with its bulging convex form that rises to a rocky crest on one side of its wide summit. Because of its proximity, it looks as large in the memoryscape as the much further away El Capitan actually is in its diorama. It reaches all the way up and fills the frame. A strip of blue sky above serves as a narrow exit point. The volcanic upthrust of the real Sanford Butte, or Circle Z Mountain, distinguishes it from the gentler hills of the Santa Ritas in which it is set. In the memoryscape, the visually intricate textures of its rocky, pock-marked surface absorb my attention. It is dotted with tall, spiked ocotillo bushes and smaller cactuses that scatter a layer of complex shadows across the ground. The scars from long, descending rock slides further mar the mountain's face. This memoryscape is difficult for me to build up and hold in place because so much of it looks similar and as a result the mountain comes into focus before me only once it is completed. The textures of the rocky slopes remind me of worn patterns in an elaborate paisley piano shawl. The shapes of the old, greening cottonwoods lining the banks of the Sonoita Creek as it snakes around the mountain's base on its way south from Patagonia to Nogales give the memoryscape a splash of color. They provide cover from the harsh sun and the massive mountain which presses down upon the creek. I find refuge and re-orientation within the spaces created among the fallen trunks strewn along the banks. The ranch sits across from the mountain above, on

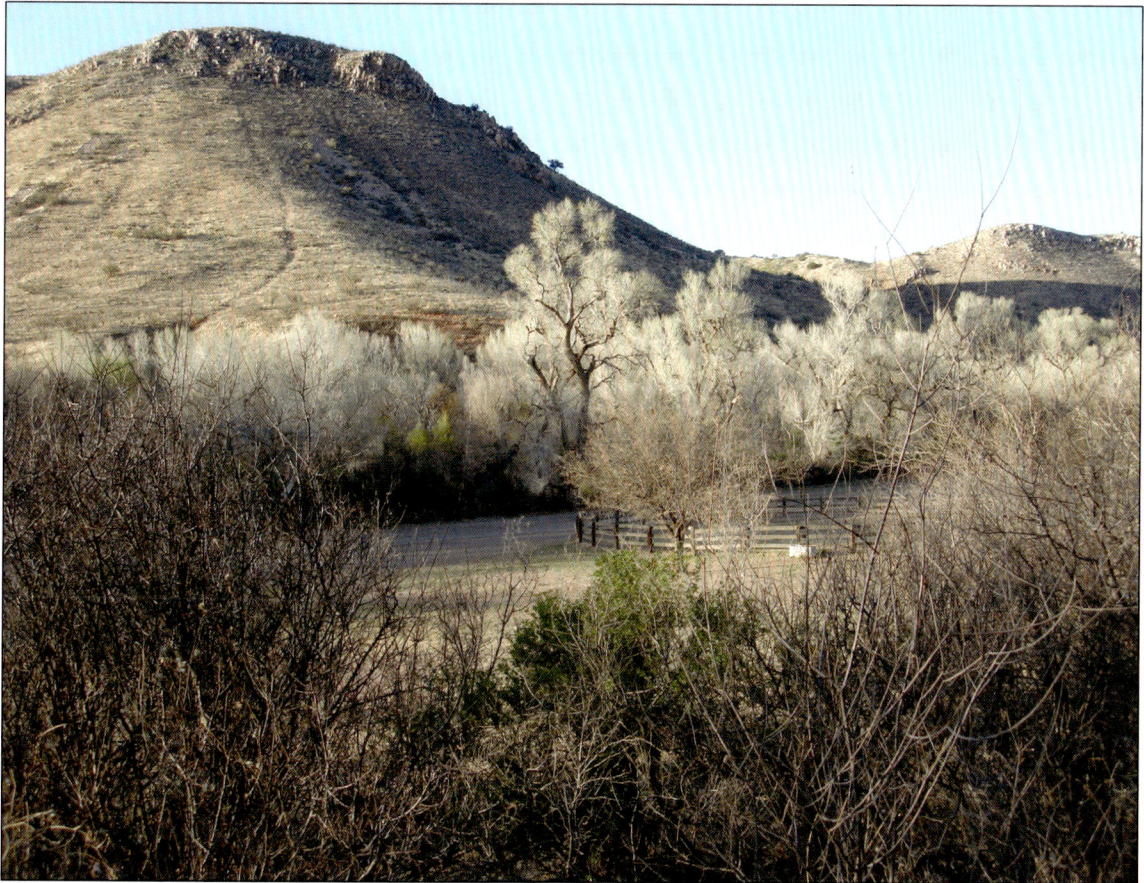

Circle Z Mountain, photograph

the other side of a field on a low ridge. It is my viewing point down into the refuge provided by the trees.

The Coyote Diorama and the Circle Z Mountain Memoryscape each showcase imposing mountains. One presents a lively midday scene, full of swirling vitality in the shadow of an immense and distant mountain; while the other presents an oddly passive and peaceful scene under a mountain that hovers close. Both the diorama and the memoryscape are credibly created places, ready to receive my glance, and both offer refuges created by the physical characteristics particular to their geography.[4]

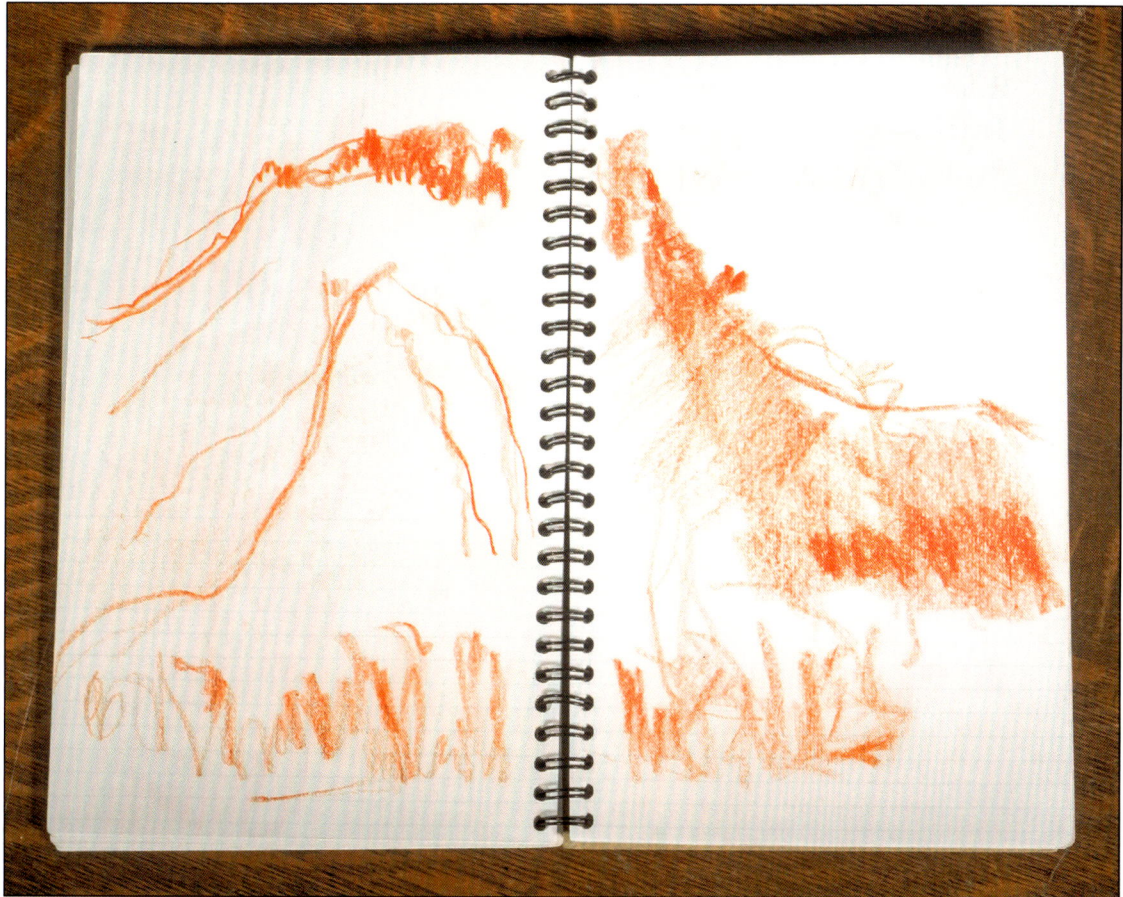

Sketch of Circle Z Mountain Memoryscape

Constance Dry

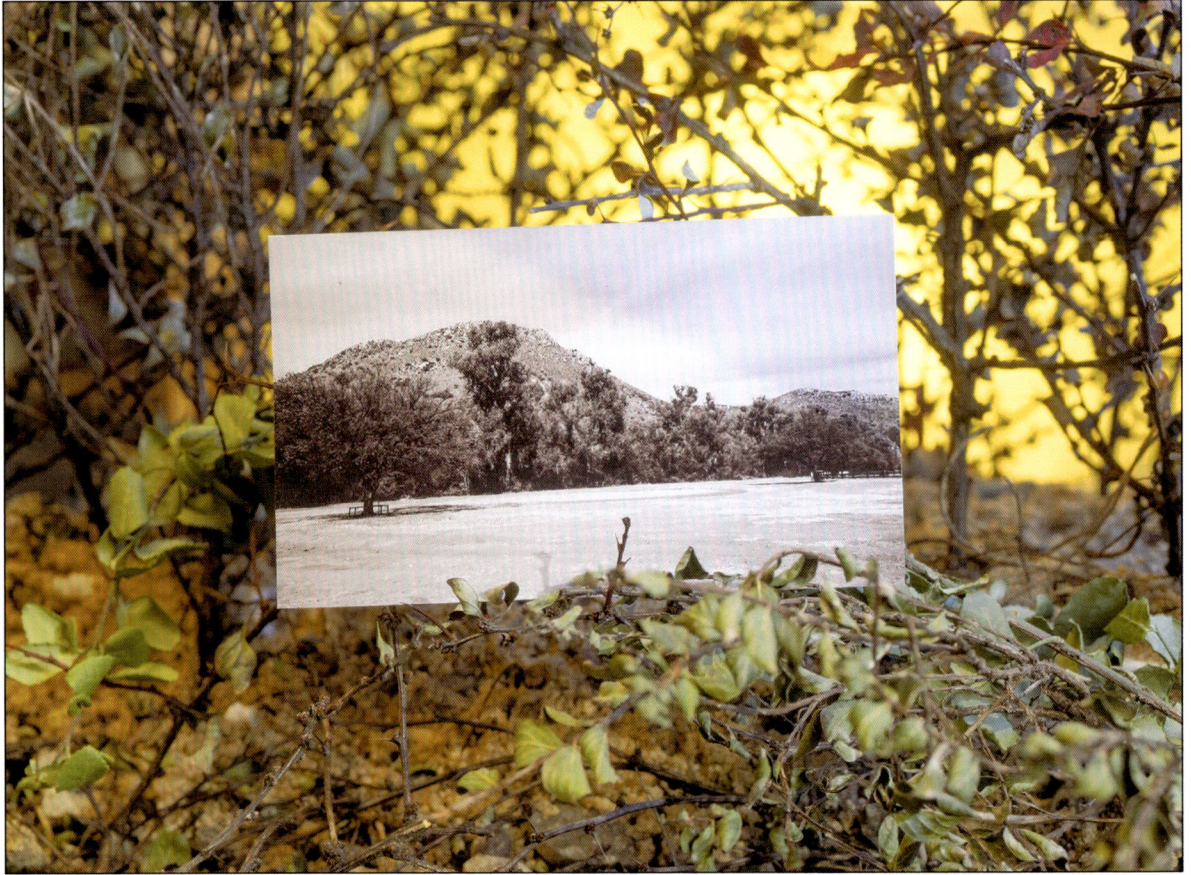

Circle Z Mountain, photograph in diorama

Justin Audet

CHAPTER SEVEN

IN SEARCH
OF CIRCLE Z

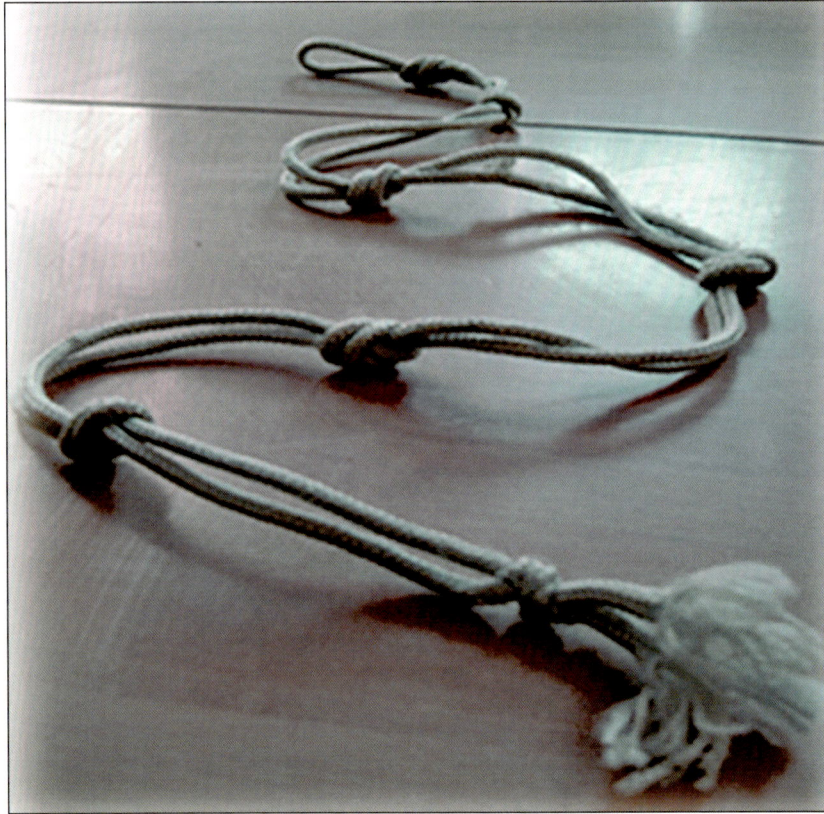

The Rope

Constance Dry

This afternoon, because of COVID, there is hardly anybody in the waiting room at the Jefferson Headache Center. Normally there is a crowd. Only a few sit here now, spaced six feet apart, all with face masks. My community of fellow patients has disappeared. I am alone again with thoughts of Mira and I wonder where she is and how she is and if her migraines have lessened. As I wait, I think about the memoryscapes and dioramas and all the medication and behavioral changes I have made during these twenty years. Migraines still create the rupture that alienates body from soul. They face each other across a seemingly unbridgeable chasm of pain, leaving me split in two and isolated from others. Only during mild attacks can I describe them. I use words like pounding, stabbing, pulsing, constricting, and unrelenting. Pain still will demand my complete attention and offer no response. Then the cycle of solipsistic absorption ensues and diminishes the world around me. Telling others about it only ricochets the pain back at me. Memoryscapes and dioramas rescue me by sidestepping all this. The chasm seals up. I feel whole again.

My searching was never for memoryscapes. They were gifts. The memoryscapes may have existed somewhere in my subconscious, but I was not aware of them in my conscious memory until the moment that they suddenly came to me. It was only once they came that they began to exist as a regular part of my consciousness. The searching I did do was a response to the effects on my soul of the presence of that terrifying void. The void impelled me to flee and search for another place that I found within the memoryscapes. I felt as if my body were a gyroscope spinning out of control, enveloped by the blackness, lost in formless space, condemned to remain there in a state of mortal fright. Only when anchored on visually stable earth with all its particulars could I regain the cardinal points of north, south, east, and west.

Imagination is not something one searches for. It arises. I had no place for a present to occur in those lost moments between past and future, no ground was available to me to stand on as a foundation for thought or imagination. The comforting real landscapes of Circle Z and the imagined memoryscapes led me farther afield to other landscapes depicted in the dioramas. Once found, they led to looking deeper. To imagine while looking is nothing new. It is done all the time. Every day, children do it when they imagine this as that through play. Understanding the content of memoryscapes as neither exclusively internal or external but dual allowed me to be in a world that was an aesthetic and psychic space as well as an actual place. We all dream or daydream or play as we experience one thing as another while it remains itself. This world amending quality of the memoryscapes healed the broken relationship between my body and soul, even as they allowed the boundaries between the real and the imagined to blur. This they share with dioramas. Both depict scenes from the natural, external world and then allow imaginary experiences to coexist within them. These interior spaces function not as rents in the fabric of reality but rather as additional layers. They open up open spaces for rich imaginative experience. These spaces became containers where memory and imagination re-emerged once I reoriented myself. The void I escaped was replaced by a feature-full place on this familiar engaging earth which I was able to experience as both this and that simultaneously.

The Circle Z I found at the end of my search was a new place with its own *genius loci*. Unlike the actual ranch, it had expanded to become the source of much healing, healing that occurred in a sphere where the real and the imagined were nourished together.

At times I would make the crowded journey from Philadelphia to New York in search of new encounters with dioramas. In sensible shoes and carrying a light backpack, I would board the Amtrak train and sit looking out the window, down at the back of the Philadelphia Zoo abutting the tracks below with its open-air habitats and live animals. Just beyond, I passed through Philadelphia's jarring vast wasteland of hulking, graffiti-tagged factory shells, a disquieting prelude to the northerly journey through New Jersey until Liberty Tower came into view, outlined against the New York skyline. Once in the bowels of Penn Station I would emerge among the sweaty crowds and take the subway up Manhattan from 34th street to the museum at 81st. Traveling this way always put me in mind of the anticipatory excitement of the early twentieth-century urban diorama viewer. She also arrived at the museum from the crowded city to view a depiction of expansive nature, untouched by man, portrayed in non-threatening, romanticized purity. For the price of admission, the dioramas would have provided, even amidst the crowded museum, a spiritual respite from city life, just as they now do for me. The taxidermied mounts behind the glass are never portrayed in the act of predation; the backdrop landscapes omit the ravages of human civilization and climate change that scar the landscape. Nature in these preserved moments is presented as benign and majestic. When the noise of New York's traffic and the motion of the busy streets makes stepping off a curb too disorienting for my migraine-ridden mind and body, the dioramas allow me to be in a place where I can linger and thrive. These gleaming jewels beckon every viewer to enter and be elsewhere. Each experience is fresh, as each viewing offers something new to see.

These days when I think of the ranch, I sometimes think of it as the second one of a slightly mismatched pair of stereopticon slides; one side retains the stain of the original landscape while the other is pitted from changes in the contemporary landscape. The cowboy myth with its reassuring dude life has faded on that side too; Circle Z as a dependable earthly retreat with its unchanging geography has buckled at the edges. Even though the actual sites of the memoryscapes have been altered in this way, as images, the memoryscapes still are radiant and the protected spaces within them are intact.

Dioramas take me from their exterior landscapes to the private space of their enclosed imagined refuges. Memoryscapes exist as private spaces that are grounded in actual public spaces. On a virtual reality headset, however, what one sees is usually not a place well known to the viewer. It often looks like an iconic but generic place that is recognizable to the viewer as a comfortable space in which to move about. Virtual reality may be very useful in the treatment of migraine pain. The sense of relief the viewer has as she moves through the sights of the virtual world before her may produce the same effect I have experienced when the neuronal pathways of pain in my brain have been diverted by looking deeply into a diorama or memoryscape. I hope these viewers who look deeply when they are enveloped by virtual reality will also be able to find toe holds, as I have, that anchor them more firmly in the specific experience of a particular place in their known world.

The mission of the museum, science entwined with education, so evident in the dioramas ensures that each viewer has all that is necessary to observe and keep observing, allowing her accumulated gazes to always yield more to see and more to know. Looking, then re-grounding, then moving on into novel experience, all began for me with a flight and a search. The search led me to view landscapes with a sustained gaze, and developing that ability has freed my body from pain and enlivened my mind with new sights, sights which are seen by viewers of the dioramas every day.[1]

✺

St. Jerome
in His Study

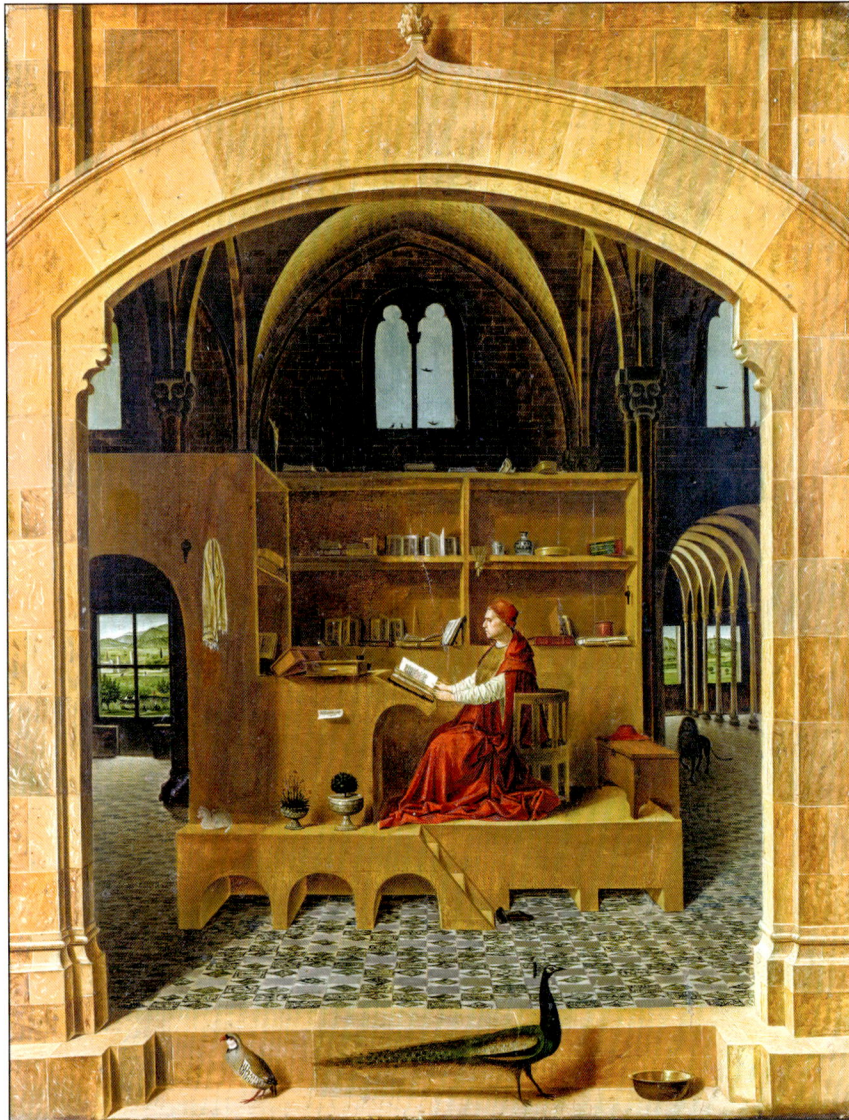

St. Jerome in His Study by Antonello da Messina

W hen I gaze at this small religious painting by Antonello da Messina, *St. Jerome in His Study*, painted around 1475, I view it with a secular eye. Seen this way, it vividly illustrates how the dioramas I visit are refuges in themselves.

The painting is itself a diorama-like vast interior landscape from which views of the outside world are glimpsed. In the immediate foreground, a wide, late-Gothic stone archway resembles the entrance to a church or a monastery. Inside, St. Jerome sits at his desk on a raised wooden structure built to look like a study carrel. Behind him, a partially enclosed wooden cubby is lined with shelves containing books and many religiously significant objects. He looks down at the brightly illuminated page of the book he holds open. The light that falls on this book, his hands, and his white undershirt is the focal point of the painting. He and this large cell-like structure completely fill the foreground of the immense space. Light enters it from four sources: the front arched opening; two mullioned windows in the rear, visible on each side of the carrel; three partially obscured trefoil windows high above; and light dramatically reflected off a series of arched colonnades placed before the rear windows on the right. Areas of alternating darkness and light fill the scene and give it a mystic airiness and contemplative calm. In linear perspective, the precisely drawn mosaic tiles begin in the foreground and extend back to the two ground floor windows to suggest the depth of this space. Pools of light fall on the tiles below the windows. Above it all, soaring interior arches create further subdivisions, suggesting other enclosed spaces.

St. Jerome sits within this imposing interior. His carrel is a refuge from distraction and danger in a space that is itself a sanctuary; the monastery. Like a diorama in the Akeley Hall, this building is its own magnificent place, a complete environment. The rays of light falling on St. Jerome re-enforce the central linear axis of the painting, and once focused on him we then look up at what surrounds him to absorb the landscape that extends from edge to edge and skyward. Its soaring arches, its alcoves and suggested rooms, extend its length and height to fill the frame. Most engaging is how the outside world is accessible to the inside. Swallows rendered in minute detail soar in the late summer afternoon light, high up outside the trefoil windows. They rest and walk along the sills. At ground level, visible through a window at the rear of the space, Antonello da Messina has painted a detailed landscape of his native Messina. Figures row along a river. A walled city is visible. A flock of sheep moves in the distance and a mountainous landscape rises above the fields under a blue sky. In the window to the right, the landscape looks more like the countryside of his Roman patrons for whom he may have intended the painting. Daylight and darkness exist side by side in the interior, each playing a part to intertwine a world of activity with a world of contemplation.

It is as if I am looking at myself at work when I look at St. Jerome. We are quite different, I know: St. Jerome seeks knowledge and communes with the divine; I seek freedom from pain to observe and imagine. He is surrounded by the objects that give religious meaning to his life: open books, manuscripts, and vessels, all arrayed on the shelves around him. But seeing him in his enclosed space reminds me that I am part of a wider sphere of those who search and seek. The permeation of the outside world into this august space sets me wondering if I too might wander more freely in the outer world and be able to incorporate some of the protective elements of refuge without the need of so much enclosure and still remain safe. Standing outside the painting, viewing it from the arched stone entrance, I imagine myself inside as whole, surrounded by a material world in which light and darkness are not at war with each other. There will always be that dip into darkness that a migraine precipitates, but equally true is the light that potential work promises. Who is to say which has the upper hand.

St. Jerome is safe at work within the secluded space of his carrel, which is within the protected space of the darkened monastery. His work so brightly illuminated by a shaft of light coming from the outside suggests to me that not only daylight interpenetrates that restricted space but knowledge of the world as well. His mind and his soul must range far beyond those muted confines. The parallel play that viewing a diorama encourages in me, during which the world can be understood and experienced as both this and that, is its own kind of meaningful work, just as are St. Jerome's tasks. Then, within the safe confines of an interior refuge, freed-up observation allows me to produce connections and realizations that then may go on to assume other forms, whether written, verbal, or imagistic. It turns out that the more focused this activity is, the more beneficial it becomes for migraine pain and the more fruitful it is as a way to understand how images work for us. Memoryscapes were the powerful engines of production that initiated all this unexpected journey.

NOTES

CHAPTER ONE: IN THE MUSEUM

1. A.E. Parr. "The role of natural history museums in the life of man." In *Natural History Museums and the Community.* Stockholm, 1969, p. 62.

2. As I note in the opening paragraph, when looking at a diorama, one of the most common responses of viewers is to ask, "Is it real?" This response was referred to in many descriptions of habitat dioramas I read. Throughout this book the distinction between realness and reality finds its way into each chapter when I attempt to compare the similarities and differences between memoryscapes and dioramas.

   My understanding of habitat dioramas in the American Museum of Natural History was shaped by the work of both Stephen Christopher Quinn and Karen Wonders. Their descriptions of the dioramas in the museum are the main source of information about them in this book. See:

   Quinn, Stephen Christopher. *Windows On Nature: The Great Habitat Dioramas of the American Museum of Natural History.* American Museum of Natural History, New York, 2006

Wonders, Karen. *Habitat Dioramas: Illusions of Wilderness in Museums of Natural History.* Uppsala University, 1993.

I have also relied on the following sources to help enrich my visits to the museum:

Poliquin, Rachel. *The Breathless Zoo: Taxidermy and the Cultures of Longing.* Penn State University Press. University Park, Pennsylvania, 2012.

Carlisle, G. Lister, Jr. "The Lion Group and Its Creation." *The Complete Book of the African Hall.* American Museum of Natural History, New York, 1936.

Casey, Edward S. *Getting Back Into Place: Toward A Renewed Understanding of the Place-World.* Indiana University Press, Bloomington and Indianapolis, 2009

CHAPTER TWO: IN THE MOVIE THEATER

1. In reflecting on my experience in the movie theater I turned to the following sources:

Brann, Eva. *Feigning: On the Origins of Fictive Images.* Paul Dry Books. Philadelphia, Pennsylvania, 2022.

Friedberg, Anne. *The Virtual Window: From Alberti to Microsoft.* The MIT Press, Cambridge, Massachusetts, 2006.

Schiecke, Konrad. *Historic Movie Theaters in Illinois 1883–1960.* McFarland Company, 2020.

Sugimoto, Hiroshi. *Theaters.* Damiani Editore/Matsumoto Editions, Bologna and New York, 2000.

In addition to nineteen years of education as a patient at the Jefferson Headache Center, my understanding of migraine was aided by the following sources:

Bourke, Joanna. *The Story of Pain: From Prayer to Painkillers.* Oxford University Press, 2014.

Foxhall, Katherine. *Migraine: A History.* Johns Hopkins University Press, Baltimore, 2019.

Milton, John. *Paradise Lost.* Macmillan Publishing Company, New York, 1993.

Llinás, Rodolfo R. *I of the Vortex: From Neurons to Self.* The MIT Press, Cambridge, Massachusetts, 2001.

Sacks, Oliver. *Migraine.* Vintage Books, Random House Inc., New York, 1999.

———. *The Man who Mistook His Wife for a Hat and other Clinical Tales.* Harper and Row, New York, 1987.

Bell, Laura. "Head Agony: Jumpy cells may underlie migraine's sensory storm." *Science News*, Vol. 181, No. #2, January 28, 2012.

Young, William, MD, and Stephen D. Silberstein, MD. *Migraine and Other Headaches.* American Academy of Neurology, Demos Health, New York, 2004.

CHAPTER THREE: AT THE RANCH

1. For a description of Roosevelt's friendship with the Eaton brothers, see the website of The Dude Ranchers Association: *www.duderanch.org.*

2. For a history of Circle Z Ranch, see their website, *www.circlez.com.* I also benefited from conversations with Diana Nash and Jennie and George Lorta.

3. For additional historical information about Patagonia and Circle Z Ranch, see:

Corkill, Gail Waechter. *Circle Z Guest Ranch.* Arcadia Publishing, Charleston, South Carolina, 2016.

Patagonia Area Resource Alliance (PARA), *www. patagoniaalliance.org.*

4. My effort to define the special meaning Circle Z has for me was aided by the following sources:

Casey, Edward. S. *Remembering: A Phenomenological Study*. Indiana University Press, 2000.

———. *Representing Place: Landscape Painting and Maps*. University of Minnesota Press, Minneapolis, 2002.

Schama, Simon. *Landscape and Memory*. Random House, New York, 1995.

Tuan, Yi-Fu. *Space and Place: The Perspective of Experience*. University of Minnesota Press, Minneapolis, 1977.

———. *Topophilia: A study of Environmental Perception, Attitudes, and Values*. Columbia University Press, New York. 1974.

CHAPTER FOUR: MEMORYSCAPES

1. In an effort to understand the origin of memoryscapes I consulted the following sources:

Arnheim, Rudolf. *The Power of the Center: A Study of Composition in the Visual Arts*. University of California Press, Berkeley, 1988.

Bachelard, Gaston. *The Poetics of Space*. Translated by Maria Jolas. Penguin Books, New York, 1964.

Brann, Eva T. H. *The World of the Imagination: Sum and Substance*. Rowman and Littlefield Publishers, Inc., 1991.

Blau, Nealy. *Elsewhere*. Decode Books. Seattle, Washington. 2011.

Casey, Edward S. *The World At A Glance*. Indiana University Press, Bloomington, 2007.

———. *Remembering: A Phenomenological Study*. Indiana Press, Indiana Press, Bloomington, 2000.

Gombrich, E.H. *The Image and the Eye: Further Studies in the Psychology of Pictorial Representation*. Phaidon Press Limited, Oxford, 1982.

CHAPTER FIVE: NEAR GUAYMAS

1. The following sources provided information about the Jaguar Diorama:

Anderson, Michael Ralph. *Painting Actuality: The Diorama Art of James Perry Wilson*. Mikey, 2019.

Anderson, Michael. James Perry Wilson: Shifting Paradigms of Natural History Diorama Background Painting, p.67 in Tunnicliffe, Sue Dale and Annette Scheersoi, ed. *Natural History Dioramas: History, Construction and Educational Role*. Springer, 2015.

Quinn, Stephen Christopher. *Windows On Nature: The Great Habitat Dioramas of the American Museum of Natural History*. American Museum of Natural History, 2006.

Northern Jaguar Project, at *www.northernjaguarproject.org*.

Sky Island Alliance, at *www.skyislandalliance.org*.

Wonders, Karen. *Habitat Dioramas: Illusions of Wilderness in Museums of Natural History*. Uppsala University, 1993

CHAPTER SIX: AT YOSEMITE

1. AMNH 57th Annual Report, July 1955–1956.
2. Sellers, Charles Coleman. *Mr. Peale's Museum: Charles Willson Peale and the First Popular Museum of Natural Science and Art*. W.W. Norton and Company, 1980, p.26.
3. Ibid., p.22.
4. Again, I owe a special debt to Stephen Quinn and Karen Wonders for their comprehensive descriptions of the habitat dioramas and their history, cited above.

   In addition, I relied on these sources for the history of habitat dioramas and Akeley's vision for the Hall:

Akeley, Carl E. *In Brightest Africa*. Garden City Publishing Co., Garden City, New York, 1925.

Barnes, John. *Precursors of the Cinema: Shadow-graphy, Panoramas, Dioramas, and Peep-shows Considered in Their Relation to the History of Cinema*. Barnes Museum of Cinematography, St. Ives, Cornwall, 1967.

Asma, Stephen T. *Stuffed Animals and Pickled Heads: The Culture and Evolution of Natural History Museums*. Oxford University Press, Oxford, 2001.

Crary, Jonathan. *Techniques of the Observer: On Vision and Modernity in the Nineteenth Century*. The MIT Press, Cambridge, Massachusetts, 1990.

Kunhardt, Peter W., Philip B. Kunhardt, JR, and Philip B. Kunhardt III. *P.T. Barnum: America's Greatest Showman*. Knopf, 1995.

Oettermann, Stephan. *The Panorama: History of a Mass Medium*. Zone Books, New York, 1997.

Sellers, Charles Coleman. *Mr. Peale's Museum: Charles Willson Peale and the First Popular Museum of Natural Science and Art*. W.W. Norton and Company, 1980.

CHAPTER SEVEN: IN SEARCH OF CIRCLE Z

1. In my search for places of refuge from the void, I wandered the byways of my memory aided by the following sources:

Bachelard, Gaston. *The Poetics of the Space*. Penguin Books, New York, 1958.

Calvino, Italo. *Invisible Cities*, translated by William Weaver. Harcourt Brace Jovanovich, 1978.

Davenport, Guy. *The Geography of the Imagination: Forty Essays*. North Point Press, San Francisco, 1981.

———. *Objects On A Table: Harmonious Disarray in Art and Literature.* Counterpoint, Washington, D.C., 1998.

Dickinson, Emily. *The Complete Poems of Emily Dickinson.* Edited by Thomas H. Johnson. Poem 419. "We Grow Accustomed to the Dark," p 200. Little, Brown and Company, Boston, 1960.

Frost, Robert. "Directive." *Steeple Bush.* Henry Holt & Co., NY, 1947.

Lucretius. *On the Nature of Things.* Book Four. Translated by Martin Ferguson Smith. Hackett Publishing Company, Indianapolis, 2001.

Shattuck, Roger. *Proust's Binoculars: A Study of Memory, Time and Recognition in A la recherche du temps perdu.* Princeton University Press, Princeton, 1962.

ACKNOWLEDGMENTS

Migraine is the backstory of this book, but it is the care I have received for my migraine disease that made the writing of it possible. I am especially in debt to the following people who have continuously provided my care from the very beginning in 2004: Dr William Young, MD, FAAN, FAHS, FANA, FCPP; Ji H. Cho, CRNP; Carla Allizo, RN; Margaret Pendergast, RN; Diane Plunkett, RN; Beth Janyszek, RN; and Terry Hasson, RN (in memoriam). Their medical attention, persistence, and inventiveness in always coming up with a plan of medication has enabled me to live a fuller life. I am also grateful to Shirley Kessel for her guidance and invaluable conversations about migraine.

Many thanks to Barbara Ciega, who began my education about dioramas and encouraged me to pursue the comparison between memoryscapes and dioramas. Her initial conversations directed my research and fueled my interest. Thank you to Mai Reitmeyer, research librarian at the American Museum of Natural History (AMNH), for assisting me in research on the Jaguar Diorama and on the work of James Perry Wilson. Tanu Naimpally of AMNH arranged an early morning visit to the museum and accompanied me on other visits. My discussion with Michael Lewis enlarged my understanding of the use of linear perspective in three-dimensional dioramas.

Thank you to Diana Nash and Jennie and George Lorta, who generously shared the history of Circle Z with me, and to my sisters, Barbara Boger and Judy Smith, whose memories provided additional information about our childhood there. In addition, Vincent Pinto supplied information about the Santa Ritas and the Patagonias to explain the natural history of the area around Circle Z. Emily Burns of the Sky Island Alliance supplied information and updates about the re-appearance of jaguars north of the border in the Sky Islands.

I am especially grateful to the following people who aided in the organization of the manuscript as well as commented on it: Ralph Zigraph, Aimee Koran, Elizabeth Begosh, Emily Marston, and Kathy Soulliere.

I owe a great deal to Justin Audet who patiently assembled and edited my photographs. He helped construct the dioramas as well as photographed them. In addition, he made a special trip to the AMNH to re-photograph dioramas, many of which made the final cut. Justin had a decisive impact on the final selection of photographs and was a great pleasure to work with. Thank you also to Brookes Britcher, August Lilley, and

Mike Kihn, who also participated in the photographing and construction of the dioramas.

From the beginning when I first mentioned the strange appearance of the memoryscapes, Eva Brann encouraged me to pursue my interest in their nature. Her book *The World of The Imagination* has been a rich source of education about images and the imagination. Its teachings about visual perception have found their way into every chapter.

I am grateful to Dr. Elizabeth Kuh for her steadfast support.

Paul Dry, as publisher, accepted the manuscript and encouraged me to be true to the experience that led to my desire to write about it. Julia Sippel, my editor, made it so much better. Thank you as well to Mara Brandsorfer and Maude de Moll Kushto of Paul Dry Books.

My husband, Paul Dry, and my daughters, Sarah and Katie, are the supportive and loving anchors of my life. They are the interlocutors who enliven me every day.